CANCER
Increasing Your Odds
for Survival

About the Author

David Bognar is an independent producer and writer who has worked for over fifteen years as a researcher and video professional. He is experienced in creating concepts, researching, scripting, producing, and editing a wide range of video and writing projects, including documentaries and local television shows. Recently he was the associate producer and editor for a one-hour documentary called *Voices,* produced in association with Connecticut Public Television, and he produced the videotape *Healing/ Dying: An Interview with Stephen Levine.*

Mr. Bognar has been employed as a researcher in a variety of positions, including paralegal work at the Hartford Institute for Criminal and Social Justice. He was also a treatment coordinator at an intermediate-level treatment facility for substance abuse, and is co-author of the book *Human Operators Manual: How Feelings Work, a Psychological Primer.*

Since the loss of his partner to breast cancer, Mr. Bognar has devoted himself to researching cancer therapies and creating the documentary and book *Cancer: Increasing Your Odds for Survival.* Information on ordering a copy of the four-part public television series narrated by Walter Cronkite, and related materials, is available at the back of this book.

Ordering

Trade bookstores in the U.S. and Canada please contact:

Publishers Group West
1700 Fourth Street, Berkeley CA 94710
Phone: (800) 788-3123   Fax: (510) 528-3444

Hunter House books are available at bulk discounts for textbook course adoptions; to qualifying community, healthcare, and government organizations; and for special promotions and fundraising. For details please contact:

Special Sales Department
Hunter House Inc., PO Box 2914, Alameda CA 94501-0914
Tel. (510) 865-5282   Fax (510) 865-4295   e-mail: marketing@hunterhouse.com

Individuals can order our books from most bookstores or by calling toll-free
1-800-266-5592

CANCER
Increasing Your Odds for Survival

A Resource Guide for Integrating
Mainstream, Alternative and
Complementary Therapies

David Bognar

Hunter House
PUBLISHERS

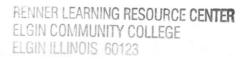

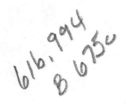

Hunter House Inc., Publishers
P.O. Box 2914
Alameda CA 94501-0914

Library of Congress Cataloging-in-Publication Data

Bognar, David.
Cancer : increasing your odds for survival / David Bognar.
p. cm.
Includes bibliographical references and index.
ISBN 0-89793-248-X (hardcover). — ISBN 0-89793-247-1 (alk. paper)
1. Cancer—Popular works. 2. Cancer—Alternative treatment. I. Title.
RC263.B59 1998
616.99'4—dc21 98-34440
CIP

Project credits

Cover Design: Jil Weil Designs   Book Design: *Qalagraphia*
Photo Credits: India Blue (David Bognar), Steve Friedman (Walter Cronkite)
Project Editor: Kiran Rana   Production Coordinator: Wendy Low
Development and Copyediting: Marianna Cherry, Priscilla Stuckey
Editorial Assistance: Belinda Breyer, Jennifer Huffaker, Jennifer Lea Gall
Proofreader: Lee Rappold   Indexer: ALTA Indexing
Marketing: Corrine Sahli, Susan Markey   Publicity: Marisa Spatafore
Customer Support: Christina Arciniega, Joel Irons
Order Fulfillment: A & A Quality Shipping Services
Publisher: Kiran S. Rana

Printed and Bound by Publishers Press, Salt Lake City, UT
Manufactured in the United States of America

9 8 7 6 5 4 3 2 1   First Edition

Contents

Part 2   Treatment

Part 3 Mind-Body Interventions

Part 4   Spirituality and Mortality

[All interviews excerpted in this book have been edited for length and clarity.]

Dedication

For people dealing with cancer

In memory of Cindy Parillo

Acknowledgments

My deep appreciation to all my friends and family who have supported me in this project these many years, including but not limited to: Paul Cimino, Mary Jane Watson, Jean Gaylord, Tom Cavagnero, Kathleen Ipacs, James Diaz, and Stephanie Mastropietro; the folks who provided me with information, like Marion Morra of the Yale Comprehensive Cancer Center, Jan Guthrie of the Health Resource, Susan Sperry of ECaP, and Frank Weiwel at People Against Cancer; Fred D'Angelo for his unfailing friendship and support; Elizabeth Beyrer for her help and editing assistance; Walter Cronkite for participating in the project; Stephen and Ondrea Levine for their loving hearts; my brother Phil for his unerring support and commitment; my new partner, Mini, for her consistent love and good cheer; and especially for the eternal Love that I believe resides in all of us.

Foreword

by R. Michael Williams, M.D., Ph.D.

It is a true honor to be invited to write this foreword for an extraordinary guide through the journey that faces every cancer patient and family member. This book accompanies a television series of the same name, and if the quality of the production comes even close to that of this exceptional guide, I can recommend this series to every cancer patient, family member, and cancer care team at every hospital in the country.

Bognar experienced the battle against breast cancer as waged by his partner, Cindy. While the cancer ultimately was never cured, the battle was fought bravely, passionately, and most importantly with attention to all possible information—the key to empowering patients and their loved ones to take control of this disease.

In the first part, cancer is described in clear, understandable terms. Statistics for survival rates are given for most of the common cancers. "Dealing with Cancer" includes the importance of second opinions, multidisciplinary settings, the types of biopsies, support services, information resources, and advice on how to deal with your doctor, your hospital, and your insurance company. Abundant references to books, Internet sites, research services, and cancer treatment organizations are described.

Bognar covers conventional therapy in adequate detail for most any layperson. A section on breast cancer even includes such topics as timing of surgery to optimize survival according to the menstrual cycle, types of surgery, predictive testing, circadian timing of chemotherapy, and a most important topic: how to deal effectively with the side effects of chemotherapy.

Patients often find that their cancers are treated as if they were the "average" cancer of that particular organ. This happens despite the fact that there are now several very well-documented studies showing the value of predictive testing of sensitivity to chemotherapy. A tumor can be obtained in the viable state and shipped under the right conditions to one of several laboratories. Bognar describes how this can be done. Would you rather have your cancer treated as if it were "average," when you could get treatment with drugs that are proven to be more likely to work? I doubt it. In fact, for most cancers that respond poorly to chemotherapy in phase II trials, drugs that do not work in the laboratory almost never work in the patient.

The information on alternative treatments really shines. Bognar even describes the AMAS test and other somewhat controversial approaches to the cancer problem. Even though the conventional oncology community may never accept these things, patients do hear about them and will welcome Bognar's clear and unbiased description. Among the alternative therapies described are 714-X, the Burzynski antineoplaston therapy, the Kelly/Gonzales program, Gerson therapy, and more esoteric treatments like Iscador, immune stimulation with placental tissue, and even the study of energy medicine.

Many medicines are developed in foreign countries. Sometimes, years elapse before the FDA approves an effective therapy so that it is readily available to physicians and patients in the United States. You should know that there is a mechanism for compassionate use by individual patients of approved medicines from foreign countries. This process is complicated. Cooperation by the physicians and the staff of the hospital, including the Investigational Review Board, often takes days of administrative work. However, an aggressive patient or patient advocate can navigate and harness this process. Bognar describes how to do just that.

Nutritional approaches as adjuvant treatment for cancer used to be outside conventional oncology. This is no longer the case. Few oncologists doubt the value of adjuvant nutrition in cancer treatment. And almost no one argues with the importance of proper nutrition to avoid cancer. Bognar even describes the use of more controversial methods such as detoxification regimens and several alternative therapies. His description of complementary or alternative medical therapies includes some widely described methods such as shark cartilage, immune stimulants, and herbs. Although this section of necessity goes into less detail on a wider range of topics, you can learn about astragalus, green tea, ginseng, and essiac tea. He also touches on acupuncture, massage therapy and oxygen treatments. I neither endorse nor condemn these methods, but remain a skeptic. Nevertheless, it is valuable to hear about them in a concise and responsible way.

This book is about a journey, one that must be taken by every cancer patient and everyone who cares about him or her. Each of us could describe our own cancer journey. David Bognar used his considerable skills in psychology and journalism to produce the TV series and this guide. My own journey started when, at thirteen years of age, my father died of small cell lung cancer. The first book I read was about Krebiozen, then came science, medicine, psychology, cultural issues, and philosophy throughout high school, undergraduate school, medical school, and graduate school. I thought that my expertise in genetics and immunology combined with standard medical training might help to complete this journey. Now I know there is much, much more to learn and to do. This guide has helped me. And I am sure that it will help you too.

R. Michael Williams, M.D., Ph.D.
Senior Medical Director and Chief Medical Officer,
Cancer Treatment Centers of America
Chairman, Cancer Consulting Group

Preface

by O. Carl Simonton, M.D.

This book is a resource guide for people dealing with cancer. It brings together expert information on the physical, mental, social, and spiritual aspects of health and healing with the valuable perspective and hard-earned wisdom of representative patients. Interviews with cancer specialists allow the reader to listen in on experts discussing the latest in treatment therapies. And the feelings and experiences of patients facing cancer are explored in depth. Because it attends to both information and feelings, the book helps the reader make wise decisions using both intellectual wisdom and intuitive wisdom (the sense that something feels right for us) so that the best path to health and healing can be found.

It is physically impossible to do everything that might make us well. Simply put, there are too many reasonable treatments available. This book guides readers through the maze of options available in both mainstream and alternative or complementary therapies. We can use the information in this book to explore these options in a way that is compatible with who we are as human beings, and to find the treatments that we can embrace.

We influence our lives and our health at all times. At no time is this more important than when we are faced with a serious illness. When facing cancer, it is important to develop and maintain a sense of hope and trust. Hope is the belief that a desirable outcome is possible, regardless of how remote it seems. In other words, hope is the belief that I *can* get well no matter how sick I am; it is not the belief that I *will* get well. Hope needs to be protected from those who do not understand it, who are ignorant of its importance in healing and would undermine our hopefulness.

We also need to develop trust in the treatments that we are receiving so we can work with the treatments and not fight them. We need to embrace our treatments as friends and allies, helping us to get well. These and other issues of the emotions, such as learning to deal effectively with fear, anger, guilt, failure, and blame are discussed in this book. The importance of our spiritual beliefs and their role in the quality of our lives and in our physical health is also richly addressed.

A key issue we face when we are seriously ill is the question of our mortality: whether we will live or die, and how we can accept that. This can influence our choice of treatment and brings up the concept of commitment without attachment: I want to get better—but it is acceptable to me if I get worse. I want to live, for I have the following reasons to live—but I am prepared to die. If I am not prepared to die, what do I need to do today to move in the direction of being ready to die? In doing this we often become more clear about what makes life meaningful.

The interviews with well-known people who have spent years dealing with the issues faced by people with serious illness provide voices of hope, wisdom, and faith. Together, their insights can reinforce our own decisions. We read their words and find their statements connecting with our own wisdom, letting us know from this heartfelt place that this choice is right for us. Connecting with this internal response can be very important in finding our own unique path to health.

All in all, this volume represents a collection of significant information that can be helpful to all of us, and especially to those of us dealing with serious illness.

O. Carl Simonton, M.D.
Simonton Cancer Center
Pacific Palisades, California

Disclaimer

The material in this book is intended to provide a review of resources, research, and cancer-related information in order to help cancer patients determine a course of action with their healthcare professionals. Every effort has been made to provide accurate and dependable information. The contents of this book have been compiled through professional research and in consultation with medical professionals. However, healthcare professionals have differing opinions, and advances in medical and scientific research are made very quickly, and groups and organizations may move or change, so some of the information may become outdated.

Therefore, the publisher, authors, editors, and professionals quoted in the book cannot be held responsible for any error, omission, or dated material. The authors and publisher assume no responsibility for any outcome of applying the information in this book in a program of self-care or under the care of a licensed practitioner. If you have any questions about the application of the information described in this book, consult a qualified healthcare professional.

Introduction

Cindy was thirty-five years old and wanted to live a full life. When breast cancer spread to her bones, she knew the conventional treatment had not saved her. Her chances for survival were near zero. She chose an alternative program that promised better odds, but the alternative therapy had no effect. Desperate, the cancer having spread to her liver and brain, we tried a combination of conventional and alternative therapies at a Toronto cancer clinic. It was too late in the disease process. I cared for Cindy until she died on January 23, 1990.

Cindy was my friend and lover. Throughout the two years of her illness, we searched desperately for the information that might help keep her alive. Though our inner resources were depleted daily, we still had to find the strength to research information, make very difficult decisions, and deal with a medical system with a view of treatment often limited to its own therapies. We were always struggling to think of the right questions to ask and where to go to find the answers we needed. Even well-intentioned doctors had limited time to spend with us, and offered little or no information on complementary therapies.

Fortunately, I had developed excellent research skills from working as a paralegal and as researcher at a program-planning think tank. My background as a researcher was helpful, but it was still difficult to acquire information when overwhelmed with the fear and sadness that Cindy might not live. I thought about how much easier this would have been if there had been some source of information that guided people through the maze of concepts, therapies, programs, and resources pertinent to surviving cancer. An overview of relevant information would have saved us time and energy that could have been devoted to Cindy, and that could have had a direct bearing on the options she chose and possibly the outcome of her illness. At the very least, the quality of both of our lives would have been greatly improved.

This book was born after Cindy died. To help me in my own healing process, and to begin the work of sharing what Cindy and I had learned together, I immersed myself even more deeply in research on cancer. I personally funded the production of a four-hour, four-part public television series, *Cancer: Increasing Your Odds for Survival.* The thrill I experienced when Walter Cronkite agreed to narrate the series was matched only by the joy of knowing that now the project would find adequate funding and the information would flow to those who needed it most—people dealing with cancer.

I am not a doctor. I am just someone who has struggled to do all I could to help my partner survive and am reporting to you what I have learned. I do not want other patients and their families to waste precious time digging for information that is less available to them because of emotional stress or time constraints or because it is not "mainstream." This resource guide is intended to get you on the road to survival as quickly as possible, armed with state-of-the-art information. It is filled with vital knowledge that cancer patients can use in conjunction with the advice of their medical treatment teams to help them choose a treatment path that can significantly enhance their odds for surviving.

Cindy's Story

Even though this book is about hope and survival, I wish to tell you about a little about my friend Cindy in the hope that you may benefit from her experience.

Cindy, although on the surface a very energetic and happy person, maintained a wall around the feelings she did not want to experience. It was like a dark area in her body she never visited. Cindy had a habit of ending conversations about feelings as soon as they began.

We all have the ability to suppress emotions we don't want to feel. This is an essential survival tool when we are children, since strong emotions are too much for our small bodies and minds to process. We use a number of techniques to stop the natural energetic flow of feelings. Feelings, however, are electrochemical events, and interrupting their flow inhibits full expression and release. The result is that the electrochemical feeling-event is stored in the muscles and tissues of the body. It can then block the flow of other feelings and electrical nerve impulses. In many cases, according to the Eastern view of medicine, the result can be physical ailments.

Most oncologists believe that cancer is a condition that develops over many years. Some experts believe that certain cancers have a great deal to do with psychological causes. It is my opinion that the emotional and physical neglect that Cindy experienced during childhood set the stage for her cancer. Cindy had a large capacity for love, but she had not learned to love herself. I believe her experience as a little girl wondering who, if anyone, was going to take care of her, and learning how to avoid the physical wrath of a drunken father, caused her to doubt she was worthy of being loved.

Cindy's job had also taken a stressful turn. After seven years booking airline reservations, she was recommended for a management training program. Against her better judgment, she decided to make the career move. She hated it. She was not well suited for the pressures and challenges of management, but returning to the phones felt like failure, so she stuck it out, becoming more doubtful of her ability and worthiness. Cindy not only had some of the prominent characteristics associated with cancer-prone personalities, she also was subject to the type of stressful life event commonly associated with the onset of the disease.

At thirty-three, Cindy found a lump in her breast that did not go away. A biopsy revealed it was cancer. At that point we didn't know enough except to hope for the best. Cindy was given a choice between a mastectomy (removal of the breast), or a lumpectomy (removal of the tumor and surrounding area). Statistically, there was no significant survival difference between the two, so Cindy had a lumpectomy and went through a course of accompanying radiation treatment. Cindy was told that her odds of surviving five years were 70 percent. Given Cindy's otherwise good health and attitude, we naturally assumed she would fall on the success side of that 70 percent.

I suppose this was our first mistake. We thought there was nothing more to do. We went on with our lives, not thinking much about it. I gave Cindy books and encouraged her to get involved with ECaP, the Exceptional Cancer Patients Program started by Dr. Bernie Siegel, the author of *Love, Medicine & Miracles*. Cindy went to a couple of group meetings, but experiencing her feelings frightened her and she stopped.

A year passed. Cindy's mammograms continued to come back negative. All was well, until she discovered another lump. Her doctor ordered X rays.

We hoped the results would be like the first time, just localized cancer. But now the cancer had spread to Cindy's spine and liver, and her odds for survival were given as only 10 percent. (Since then I have been told by more than one physician that survival odds for metastatic breast cancer are realistically much lower.)

Cindy wanted to stay alive, and a 10 percent chance of living wasn't good enough. She wanted to go for broke—for life. We decided to see what else was out there. I was a good researcher. I knew how to find information and answers to questions, and we obtained reports specific to Cindy's cancer and stage of cancer from two research services. The Health Resource provided an excellent volume of information resources and research at a reasonable fee. At a cost of four hundred dollars, Can Help, operated by Pat Grady, a former medical journalist, provided a ten-page letter that highlighted the unconventional and conventional treatment options that his research suggested were the best ones. One of the treatments he recommended was offered by Dr. Nicholas Gonzalez in New York City.

Gonzalez's approach appealed to Cindy. It was based on supplements, health foods, and natural healing techniques—things with which she was familiar. Participating in the program was a full-time job. The schedule of enzymes, juicing, preparation, cleansing procedures, and supplements took up most of the day.

At first, although hectic, the program went relatively smoothly. I still wanted Cindy to do the psychological work, but it wasn't more than a month or so before her deteriorating physical condition made this unrealistic. But she remained faithful to the program, believing that success depended on her commitment. Then, one day, she lost consciousness.

CAT scans revealed the cancer had spread to her liver and brain. The treatment had not worked. I had read of a Dr. Scheef in Germany who had successfully treated patients with cancer that had metastasized to the brain, so we investigated further. Scheef's treatment uses an aggressive chemotherapy not available in the United States. In order to handle the chemotherapy, Dr. Scheef wanted his patient's liver to be at least 50 percent intact. Unfortunately, CAT scans revealed that tumors had replaced over 50 percent of Cindy's liver, so we went to our backup plan: the Falk Clinic in Toronto.

Rudy Falk, the chief oncologist at Toronto General, operated his own cancer clinic where he could apply more experimental treatments. He used a combination of conventional and alternative treatments and had had success in dealing with both brain and liver metastasis. It seemed like our best bet.

I remember choking back tears as I wheeled Cindy through Toronto airport. She was still engaging, with a half-paralyzed smile as she tried to keep up our spirits. I smiled a crooked grin, too. Crooked because I was afraid, and I didn't want her to see my fear and my tears. The cancer in her spine had destroyed vertebrae and her ability to walk. She was in a great deal of pain, but we had established a level of pain medication that made her comfortable and still able to communicate. For me everything was a blur of stress, decisions, and actions, with no time for feelings. This was our last chance.

For the next two weeks, every morning Cindy's sister Lisa and I wheeled Cindy into the clinic, where she received treatments until three or four every afternoon.

Then, good news. The treatment was working! The nurse showed us on ultrasound how the tumors had changed, indicating that they were dying. We were told that if the brain tumors did dissolve, normal or near-normal brain function could return. We thought we had at least bought some time and that survival was still a possibility. Unfortunately, there is a point where the body has been compromised beyond return and treatment of any sort seldom works.

The day before we were to leave, one last treatment was scheduled. Afterward, Cindy fell into a sleep, as she often did, but this time we were unable to awaken her. The staff said critical body systems were beginning to fail. The clinic was closing for the day. We tried to get her admitted to a hospital, but for various reasons, to our surprise, this was not possible. We hired a nurse to come in for the evening to help us.

And then Cindy just stopped breathing. There was this horrible stillness. Then, the realization—Cindy was dead. It was so unbelievable. The idea that she was not ever going to move again, be here again, talk to me again. It was totally incomprehensible to me that people died and were gone, never to be with us again. I realize now how naive I was, how lucky never to have lost a loved one to death until the ripe age of thirty-five.

I remember being thankful for the kind nurse. Her simple knowing presence was comforting. She had seen this before, many times. People died, and people lived on.

Cindy's healing journey ended in Toronto on January 23, 1990.

That same day marked the beginning of my healing journey, a major part of which became the making of a documentary and this book to help others with cancer.

What This Resource Guide Offers

From discussions of coping with the initial shock of diagnosis to assessments of leading mind-body therapies, this book is designed to be a comprehensive overview of topics essential to increasing survival odds. It includes treatments, complementary therapies, latest developments, commentary, organizations, and resources pertinent to surviving cancer.

This guide also contains my opinions. I am candid in my assessments because I know you don't have time to waste. You need to know what is worthy of your attention and what is not. I am committed to providing useful information in as simple and direct a manner as possible. You must judge what is relevant to your situation. Just as there are many types of cancers and causes, there are many different potential solutions. Each person has the responsibility for choosing a healing program that is best for him or her. This guide, hopefully, will make this task much less difficult.

Recently there has been a lot in the news about the development of new, more effective treatments, possibly even a cure for cancer. While progress in the search for new, effective treatments is promising, it can give people the impression that there is no need to look further. The idea that the cure we hope for is at hand can lead some people to think, "Just hang on, wait a little longer, the cure is coming." Unfortunately, the cure isn't here yet and cancer patients don't have the time to wait; they need to know what is available to help them survive now. The reality is that only a very few patients will get into clinical trials for the most promising of these treatments. There is also the disconcerting requirement of research science that some patients receive only placebos for what many believe is their last hope to live. Participating in clinical trials is a gamble, just as the use of alternative and even conventional treatments can be. Research into the effectiveness of all forms of treatment and the wise use of complementary therapies can help stack the odds in your favor.

Gathering Information

This guide has been designed to help those who want to live. It will help you make your best effort at surviving. Taking the time now to research what you can do for your cancer can save you pain, aggravation, and possibly your life. Even if some complementary therapies, like meditating or using imagery, do not appeal to you, there is much that can be done at all levels of involvement. What is important is acquiring and applying the information judiciously to deal with your specific cancer.

Some of the information may challenge the way you presently think. I recommend that you remain open to new information, yet be discerning. If you assume that you already know the truth about alternative treatments, conventional medicine, or other aspects of healing, you may deny yourself knowledge that may contain the information vital to increasing your chances of survival.

Western science is just beginning to acknowledge that our health and our bodies are part of a much more complicated interactive system affected by many factors, including our thoughts and emotions. We are beginning to see the emergence of a new medical model, a view of health and disease that is inclusive, holistic, and open to both the so-called hard and soft sciences.

This guide does not break down cancers into subspecialties of individual cancers. It is a general resource guide aimed at empowering the cancer patient and family, and it will help you choose your path to healing. It will even help you define what healing is for you. Within these pages are steps that can help you to become personally empowered to cope with your cancer diagnosis.

I have included excerpts from my interviews with cancer treatment and healing specialists. I specifically chose certain experts to represent the full spectrum of healing approaches. The interviews address theories and philosophies of the physical, emotional, spiritual, and psychological aspects of coping with cancer and finding a path to healing. These acknowledged specialists, who committed their time and energy to these interviews, spoke from their experience and their hearts.

To increase the odds of surviving cancer, there is much to do and learn. Cancer can be a cruel teacher, but for many its lessons have led to a more satisfying life and to healing beyond their expectations. I sincerely hope the information gathered here facilitates your healing journey.

Part 1

Diagnosis and Empowerment

1

Understanding Cancer

What Is Cancer?

Cancer is a condition in which an abnormal body cell mutates and multiplies uncontrollably. A normal cell is created with a set of genetic instructions telling it how to multiply, how long to live, and when to die. But due to a genetic flaw, or exposure to carcinogens, radiation, viruses, or other causes unknown, a change in the genetic message may alter those instructions and the cell multiplies out of control. At first, the mutant cells multiply slowly and are vulnerable to attacks by the immune system. Often the process accelerates, and the increasing number of cells then typically form a mass of tissue referred to as a "tumor."

There are two types of tumors, malignant and benign. Benign tumors typically do not invade "healthy" neighboring tissue and, in most cases, pose no health threat.

In a malignant tumor, cancerous cells break off and travel through the bloodstream or the body's lymphatic system. Lymphatic vessels carry lymph fluid, a yellowish, transparent fluid that transports lymphocytes, white blood cells, and other disease-fighting cells in order to cleanse the body of toxins that can burden the immune system or cause disease. Malignant cancer cells are often trapped in lymph nodes, another part of the immune system, where many of the cancer-fighting cells are located. The lymphatic system is a filtration system, keeping toxins and other matter from entering the bloodstream.

This process in which the cancerous cells travel through the body is called "metastasis." When a cancer metastasizes or spreads, cancerous cells can be lodged in a wide variety of organs throughout the body, where they can grow into new malignant tumors. As a malignant tumor grows in size, it can obstruct the proper function of the organ it occupies, eventually destroying it.

Cancer diagnosis includes an indication of how far the cancer has metastasized from where it began. The "stages" of cancer, as they are called, differ only slightly from cancer to cancer. Stage one is usually when the cancer is "local" or has not spread. Stage two cancer, also called an intermediate or regional stage, is when the tumor has spread, usually to lymph nodes that are nearby. Stage three, or advanced, cancer is when the cancer has spread to distant parts of the body remote from where the cancer began.

Five-Year Survival Rates

People are considered to have recovered from cancer if they are still alive five years after diagnosis. These are called five-year survival rates. Five-year survival rates are sometimes thought of and presented as the percentage of people that are cured of cancer, but this is not always true. As Dr. Albert Marchetti explains in the interview below, since it is hard to track patients over a lifetime, the span of five years was chosen as a reasonable amount of time in which to gather data. The statistics may include people who are alive but not necessarily cancer free, since recovery is measured by survival, not by absence of cancer cells in the body.

Five-Year Relative Survival Rates by Stage at Diagnosis

Site	All Stages	Local %	Regional %	Distant %
Oral	53	81	42	18
Colon-rectum	62	93	67	8
Rectum	60	88	55	5
Pancreas	4	15	5	2
Lung	14	49	18	2
Melanoma	88	95	61	16
Female Breast	84	97	76	21

Cervix uteri	69	91	49	9
Endometrium (uterus)	84	96	66	27
Ovary	46	93	55	25
Prostate	89	100	94	31
Urinary	81	94	49	6
Kidney	59	88	60	9
Liver	6	13	7	2

(American Cancer Society. Cancer Facts and Figures—1998. Atlanta, GA: American Cancer Society, 1998. Booklet.)

The General Accounting Office (GAO) has said that many of the apparent advances in cancer are statistical—due to an increase in finding cancer sooner. Earlier discovery puts more people in the five-year-survival-rate window. Take breast cancer, for example. The GAO reported that for one period studied, the five-year survival rate had gone up, but mortality, or the number of women dying, had remained the same.

Booklets

Cancer Facts and Figures—1998, from the American Cancer Society (listed in the white pages), and *Cancer Rates and Risks,* from the National Institutes of Health (1-800-4-CANCER). Free publications showing five-year survival rates for your specific cancer and stage are available from your physician or by calling 1-800-4-CANCER (1-800-422-6237) with your exact diagnosis.

Knowing Your Odds

Many people prefer not to know their survival odds. On one level this makes sense. They are only statistics. You can be on either side of the survival statistic. Realistically, if the odds say 90 percent of people die from your cancer in five years, this can give you a fairly clear picture of how effective conventional medicines are for your cancer. It can help you make decisions about what kind of treatment to seek.

When faced with a cancer that is terminal or for which the survival odds are very low using conventional treatment, your best hopes are experimental treatments, clinical trials, and alternative and complementary therapies. Knowing where your cancer falls in the statistics can set you on the path of investigating alternatives sooner, which can increase your odds for survival.

If your survival odds are promising, it is possible to be lulled into a false sense of security. Facing the reality that your body has a propensity for cancer is difficult. It is easier to assume you will be in the percentage that survives. Although this may be the case, you can stack the odds further in your favor by doing what you can to avoid recurrence. Cancer is most deadly when it returns and metastasizes. For this reason, it is the time after initial treatment that is most wisely used to pursue options that can reduce the chance of recurrence. This guide, and the documentary series of the same name, describes many therapies to help prevent cancer from returning after initial diagnosis and treatment.

Getting Informed

Gathering information about your cancer is an important empowering activity. Your doctor and the hospital staff, no matter how good they are, have limited time, and their specialized viewpoints of treatment options often do not include complementary and alternative approaches. Knowing the questions to ask, and how to determine if you are receiving the most up-to-date treatment, can itself make a huge difference in how well your treatment works. In addition, you will experience profound benefits from having some sense of control over your treatment.

Take the time to find out your cancer and stage, your prognosis, and what is available to help you survive. This can make a significant difference in the quality of your life and in your odds for surviving cancer.

A New Medical Model

There is a revolution occurring in the way we look at disease. People now have increased access to information about many medical and healing disciplines from around the world. They are taking the best of different approaches and not limiting themselves to one model or therapy. People are also becoming better medical "consumers," understanding that doctors, no matter how well intentioned, cannot know everything in conventional or alternative medicine. There is a growing understanding that doctors are consultants who are paid for their services by the patient. Customers of health services are increasingly aware that medicine is also a business, and they have become wary of practitioners who are blindly critical of information that falls outside of their area of expertise.

You have the right, as a consumer, to choose the treatment or treatments you feel are best for your particular type of cancer. You can use conventional medicine or alternative medicine, or you can supplement one with the other. You can seek out open-minded health professionals who will provide or direct you to the type of treatment you choose. If your service provider is skilled in only one kind of medicine, conventional or alternative, you can pursue referrals to other types of treatment. Good doctors are open-minded and will encourage their patients to research, ask questions, and actively participate in their treatments. You can increase your survival odds by finding those physicians and treatments that offer the best combination of therapies for your healing.

The new synthesis of medical knowledge gleans information from a variety of medical models and health-related bodies of knowledge, old and new, from around the globe. The view of the body as an energy system is one of the most exciting elements of the emerging medical model. It views disease as a manifestation of an interruption in the flow of vital energies in the body, and sees humans as intimately connected to a larger energy system or a benevolent unified field. The potentials for healing and understanding are tremendous.

This book is intended to acquaint you with some of the information available in the new synthesis, and to help you take responsibility for understanding your disease and caring for yourself. It is the embodiment of a holistic approach, one that uses the best of every approach to help the patient. Conventional, alternative, supplemental, or a combination of several—the treatments you choose need to be the ones that are right for you. As is the case with learning about anything new, until we know more, our knowledge is incomplete. There will be misinformation, mistakes, and conflict. It is an inevitable aspect of change. This should not deter people seeking to heal themselves. A great deal of knowledge already exists and is available to those willing to make the effort. As we learn to incorporate these diverse and intriguing bodies of knowledge we will be better able to care for our needs and receive the healing benefits this approach offers.

Book

James S. Gordon, M.D., *Manifesto for a New Medicine: Your Guide to Healing Partnerships and the Wise Use of Alternative Therapies* (Reading, MA: Perseus Press, 1996).

Interview with
Albert Marchetti, M.D.

on Five-Year Survival Rates, Spontaneous Remissions, the Immune System, and Alternative Treatments

Albert Marchetti is a dedicated and compassionate pathologist, practicing in Manhattan, who wanted to help people learn about the range of hopeful therapies available to cancer patients. Early in our research, Cindy and I came across his book *Beating the Odds: Alternative Treatments That Have Worked Miracles Against Cancer.* We appreciated how informative, concise, and hopeful the book was. Unfortunately, like many good books, this one is out of print, but I was pleased to have gathered some important pieces of information in his interview.

You are a pathologist. Would you describe what cancer is?

Generally, it's a group of cells that are out of control. They grow in total disrespect of the tissue around them and invade other organs and other tissues, eventually bringing about the destruction of the body.

Define for people how "disease free" is measured in the five-year survival rate.

One of the problems of reporting cancer and one of the problems with cancer statistics is that they are reported on a five-year basis. Physicians understand what that means. They understand that if an individual is alive after five years, they are considered to be a "cure." If the individual expires one day after the five years, they are *still* considered to be a cure. Unfortunately, it is difficult to follow patients for their lifetime to determine how long they indeed live after they are diagnosed as having cancer, which is why the five-year survival rate was established.

Still, it is a point of confusion for patients, because when they are told they have a 50 percent chance of being cured, that simply means they have a 50 percent chance of living five years. A 90 percent chance of being cured means that they have a 90 percent chance of living for five years. So if the patient understands that, everything is put into perspective. But many times it's misleading.

What are spontaneous remissions? Do you believe they occur? Do people bring them on themselves?

The concept of spontaneous remission is a very important one in cancer therapy. It shows many things. It shows that the body is capable of curing its own illnesses. A spontaneous remission is a regression of cancer without treatment, without therapy, with no real explanation. Spontaneous remissions are, in a sense, mysteries. The mysterious part is that some experience them and others don't.

Why do they occur? Probably because the natural defense system of the individual is spurred. It gets stimulated and develops enough potential to overcome the cancer. In other individuals this doesn't happen, and they don't experience a spontaneous remission.

Spontaneous remissions have been documented since the turn of the century. They were first noted in Europe, in Germany, and in England. But they were then noted in the United States, and cases began appearing in the medical literature. In 1966 two American doctors did a relatively exhaustive study in which they examined the tissue and medical histories of perhaps thousands of patients and came up with a fairly large number of true, documented spontaneous remissions. They included only cases where there were tissue samples [to show] that an absolute diagnosis of cancer had been made and where the individuals received no therapy and yet were totally cured of their disease. So spontaneous remissions are indeed real.

They occur with an unknown frequency, but they probably occur much more frequently than any of us imagine. As a matter of fact, each of us probably experiences spontaneous remissions every single day. As cancer cells develop within our bodies, our natural defense systems identify them and immediately eradicate them. It's a natural phenomenon; it's something that we do constantly. When an individual is diagnosed as having cancer—cancer so overwhelming that they have symptoms—if for some reason that cancer disappears, that is the phenomenon most people think of as a spontaneous remission. But each of us experiences spontaneous remissions probably every day.

What are the conditions under which spontaneous remissions normally happen? For example, are they mostly religious in nature? Can people do something to create them? What are the circumstances or intervening factors that seem to create a spontaneous remission?

The factors that create spontaneous remissions are extremely varied. Sometimes they are associated with spiritual or religious events. Sometimes they are associated with a change of diet, sometimes with a vigorous exercise program, and sometimes they occur with no explanation whatsoever. Some people experience them with absolutely no anticipation, with absolutely no change in their daily life pattern, whereas other people experience them after they've undergone some incredible event in their life, such as a spiritual happening or a significant change in diet, a psychological change in their attitude. But in general, spontaneous remissions are unpredictable.

What are some of the natural mechanisms the body possesses to fight cancer, and what is the process of healing?

The processes of healing and the processes that bring on spontaneous remissions are normal processes of our body. From the time we are born to the time we die, our bodies are constantly in a defensive posture. We are constantly defending ourselves against viruses, bacteria, invading organisms, and also cancer cells. Our bodies have been blessed with an incredible array of cells and substances that not only *prevent* cancer but also many times *reverse* cancer once it begins.

The natural substances and cells that participate in the defense include macrophages, which are cells that wander throughout the body, traveling in the bloodstream. They leave the bloodstream and enter tissues in constant search of substances, such as cancer cells, that are considered foreign by our bodies. When macrophages come in contact with a cancer cell, they will engulf it, a process known as *phagocytosis*. They actually engulf the entire cell and then liquefy the cell within their own cellular bodies and in that way destroy cancer.

Lymphocytes are another kind of blood cell that plays a very significant role in cancer therapy and in the natural defense against cancers. Lymphocytes are geared not only to identify cancer cells, but also, when stimulated by interferon, another natural substance produced by the body, to become killer cells, attacking cancer and destroying it. Interferon is one of the [more recently discovered] substances that the body produces. It's produced by lymphocytes and also by fibroblasts, which are fiber cells. The interferon has a variety of anticancer properties, including a mechanism by which cancer cells are not allowed to migrate, and antiviral activities that prevent viruses from entering cancer cells.

So there are many natural substances that are occurring within our bodies that help us defend against cancer.

One of the more exciting areas in medicine today is recombinant technology, whereby scientists are able to clone cells and genetically engineer them so that they produce naturally occurring substances such as interferon, interleuken, perhaps tumor necrosis factor, another substance shown to be very powerful in destroying cancers. And as medical technology becomes more adept in identifying these substances and producing them, we will then be given another weapon against cancer, using the chemicals of our own bodies to fight the disease.

Going a little further into that, what is the thymus gland? Some people say that the thymus gland manufactures T cells. Is that correct?

There are a variety of organs in the body that aid in cancer defense—the bone marrow, our lymph glands, the thymus gland. The thymus gland is particularly responsible for T lymphocytes, the cells that identify cancer and become natural killer cells when influenced by interferon. They are one of the more powerful anticancer cells that we possess. The thymus gland is a relatively large gland during childhood, but it diminishes with time and with age and eventually disappears from the body completely around age sixty. Consequently, the influence of the thymus gland also diminishes with time. Perhaps this is one of the reasons why cancer seems to strike older people more frequently than younger people.

Is there any research indicating that vitamins and supplements can help a body fight cancer?

There are a number of studies that show that some foods and food substances, such as vitamin supplements, aid in cancer defense.

The most expansive and perhaps the most controversial studies were conducted by Linus Pauling. One of his more interesting works compared the longevity of individuals who had similar forms of cancer and were of similar ages. They basically fell into the same groups. He placed one hundred of these individuals on large doses of vitamin C and left one thousand of them with no vitamin therapy whatsoever. The individuals who were placed on the vitamin C lived significantly longer than those who received no vitamin therapy whatsoever.

That study has not been duplicated, but many people believe that Pauling's findings are indeed legitimate. He personally felt that if he had increased the dose of vitamin C that he gave the one hundred patients in his study, they would have lived even longer. One of the nice things about vitamin C therapy is that it has no real downside. The vitamin is not toxic. It is a water-soluble vitamin, so excesses are eliminated from the body very quickly. It's one of those components of an adjunct cancer therapy that really has much more benefit than any detriment.

One of the points I would like to discuss is the process that a patient should go through when they are identified as having cancer. I would like to put the alternative, or adjunct, therapies in perspective. I have very strong feelings about adjunct therapies. I believe they should be used in all cases of cancer.

I believe cancer therapies are divided into two main areas today: (1) the traditional therapies of course, which are surgery, chemotherapy, radiation, and hormonal therapies; and (2) adjunct therapies, also known as alternative therapies (sometimes called unorthodox therapies).

The medical community, on the one hand, is extremely concerned that individuals will participate in alternative therapies and *not* seek traditional medicine, which has [the advantage of] documented proof of effectiveness and of increased survival rates. The traditional therapies have been studied extensively, and they are very well controlled. They have been shown statistically to produce results. On the other hand, alternative therapies basically haven't been studied so well, and their effectiveness is based predominantly on testimonials. Within traditional medical communities, testimonials are not viewed as medical fact, as supportable data. Consequently, doctors in the field of traditional medicine view them almost with disdain. And many times, they'll tell patients that they are totally wasting their time by participating in a form of alternative therapy.

I, on the other hand, don't believe this is true. I think if an individual is diagnosed with cancer, that person should seek out the finest medical or surgical help they can get. If it means traveling from California to New York, then that's what they should do. They should get two opinions, and where there is conflicting information, they should get a third opinion. They should submit themselves to the therapies that statistically will provide them with the greatest chance of survival. However, after having been diagnosed and after having been treated, I think it's foolish for a person to sit on their sofa and hope that they are cured. They should participate in some form of alternative therapy that provides a goal, that provides hope, that provides faith, and that provides another chance of beating their cancer. There are a variety of alternative therapies that they can participate in, and they should pick and choose those that they feel will be most beneficial to them.

Can you distinguish among supplemental, adjunct, and alternative therapies? In what way should they be combined?

Some people make a distinction, thinking that a certain therapy should be used either as an *alternative* to traditional medicine or as a *supplement* to traditional medicine. I personally believe that they should be used as a *supplement* to traditional medicine.

I believe that fighting cancer is like running a mile race. If you had to run a mile race against five of the finest world-class milers alive, the chances are that you would lose the race; and if your life depended on winning, you would also lose your life. However, if you can place yourself fifty yards from the finish line while all the other runners had to start at the starting line, there is a good chance you would finish first, win the race, and win your life. Well, you place yourself fifty yards from the finish line by obtaining the finest medical and surgical care you can get. But you still have to cross the finish line to win the race, to save your life. And you go the extra fifty yards on your own, and you do that with the supplemental, alternative, or adjunct therapies available today.

In distinguishing among the alternative therapies, some therapists or alternative physicians believe that the alternative approach to cancer therapy is more valuable than the traditional approach. In some cases this may be true. For example, if the patient has a very advanced tumor, a very advanced malignancy, and there is very little that the traditional medical community has to offer, then the individual can turn confidently to an alternative therapy that perhaps has not been proven statistically to be of benefit. If an individual has a very advanced tumor and their physician says that it is inoperable or that the tumor is in an area that cannot be radiated, or there's no role for chemotherapy at all, that leaves the patient essentially with no alternative. Basically, the physician is saying to the patient, "You might as well go home and die."

I don't accept that, and a patient should never accept that. There are many other forms of therapy not included in the traditional armamentarium that patients can use to significantly improve their lives, extend their longevity, and perhaps bring about a spontaneous cure.

Do you think people should know the survival odds of conventional treatment for their specific stage of cancer, and if so, why?

Whenever a patient is seen by a physician, and is told they have cancer, there are a number of questions the patient should ask of the doctor. They should ask: (1) How much time do I have? (2) What kind of cancer is it? and (3) How fast is it growing? If a patient is told that her cancer is a very slow-growing cancer—for example, carcinoma of the cervix—she will know that she has a significant amount of time to make a decision. Her doctor can tell her that the normal course in this particular form of disease requires many, many years to become invasive. On the other hand, if a patient is told that he has a choriocarcinoma of the testicle, and his physician tells him how aggressive that type of cancer is, the patient must realize that he does not have a lot of time. He must make a decision quickly.

So, first we should know what kind of cancer we're dealing with. The patient should ask, "What is my diagnosis? How long does this cancer grow? How fast does it grow? How much time do I have to make a decision?" And when they're provided with that information, then they should ask what the alternative treatments are, what the statistical chances are of being cured, what the statistical chance is that they will be alive five years from now, what the chances are that they will be completely cured. There are very good statistics for most of the traditional forms of medical and surgical treatments for cancer, so the doctor should be able to give a very good projection. Once the patient has that information, then they can seek out a second opinion if they feel that they should. They can go to a larger medical center and be treated by a very competent physician. Or if they are dealing with a physician who has very good credentials and has treated that particular disease successfully, then they can stay in the care of that physician.

Cortisol is something you talk about quite a bit in your book. Could you talk a little bit about it?

Many people wonder why they got cancer. There are many causes of cancer, one of the most significant being an abnormal or weakened immune system. When we are confronted with a cancer threat, it is up to the cells and substances of our natural defense system to put things back into control. However, if the natural defense system is weakened for whatever reason, the cancer may be able to get a foothold and then grow out of control.

One of the substances of the body that weakens the natural defense system, our immune system, is cortisol, which is a steroid produced by the adrenal glands and which is often associated with chronic stress. If an individual is overly stressed for a long period of time, the immune system suffers. Cortisol is pumped out in excessive amounts and for a prolonged period of time, and the immune system is then weakened and cancer has the opportunity to grow.

One of the classic examples of how substances such as cortisol affect the immune system was very well demonstrated in a case of transplantation medicine, where an individual was given a transplant kidney and, following the operation, began to go through some of the symptoms of organ rejection. To prevent organ rejection, chemicals (i.e., drugs) such as steroids are provided so that the immune system is depressed and the organ is not rejected. (It is our immune systems that are responsible for tissue or organ rejection.) In the aforementioned patient's case, the rejection of the organ was found not to be a rejection at all, but rather the symptoms of a tumor, which had appeared in the patient's lungs and in the transplanted kidney.

This initially perplexed the doctors that were working on this case. Prior to surgery, there were no tumors in the lungs. Chest X rays had been performed, and they were completely normal. When the kidney was examined before it was transplanted into the individual, it seemed to be completely normal. The doctors working on the case then believed what had probably occurred was the growth of a cancer that was only microscopic in the kidney. But the cancer had grown because the individual had been given immunosuppressive drugs, such as cortisol. When the immune system was depressed, the cancer began to grow out of control and to spread to the patient's lungs, literally within days. When the physicians realized what was going on, the patient was taken off the immunosuppressive drugs, and the cancer immediately resolved. Of course, the kidney was rejected because that is the normal function of the immune system. So without being suppressed, the immune system began to function properly and the organ was rejected. But the good news was that the cancer spontaneously disappeared. It's an example of how suppression of the immune system supports or promotes the growth of cancer.

Now, you're talking about the immune system. So what is immunotherapy?

The thought that a competent immune system is necessary for cancer control supports the use of immunotherapies, which are therapies that stimulate the immune system. Interferon, in a sense, is an immunotherapy. It is an immune modulator, and it stimulates the immune system in a way that is detrimental to the growth of cancer. So when an individual thinks that a suppressed immune system will contribute to the growth of cancer, they are a little confused. Immunotherapies stimulate the immune system; they do not suppress the immune system.

Could you talk a little bit about the macrobiotic diet and the kind of results it's had?

One of the forms of alternative therapies is the macrobiotic diet. The rationale behind the diet is based on the recognition that foods may cause cancer. The American Medical Association and traditional medicine in the United States have become accustomed to this thought and now support the belief that excessive diets—diets that are high in fat and also calories—may contribute to the growth of cancer. There have been a number of nutritional studies done in the past, not only with animals but also on humans, to show that foods are absolutely related to the development of cancer. Post–World War II studies in Japan showed a significant increase in American forms of cancer in Japanese individuals who were placed on Americanized diets. In World War II, in the Netherlands, when individuals had to turn to grains and vegetables in place of meat and eggs because rations and food supplies were low, the incidence of cancer actually decreased. These are just two examples of how foods may contribute to the development of cancer.

The macrobiotic philosophy goes one step further: not only do foods contribute to the development or growth of cancer, but also a modification of diet can actually reverse the tendency, can actually put cancer in check, and can actually bring about remissions. The statistical proof of this form of therapy is weak. There have not been any well-controlled placebo studies that are double-blind and are acceptable in terms of traditional medical scientific standards and that support the use of macrobiotics in the treatment of cancer.

However, I personally believe that any therapy—regardless of whether it's nutritional or spiritual or visual—that can change the environment within us can have a very beneficial effect and can stem the cancer tide. Cancer cells, in a sense, are weak cells. They are devoid of many of the structures that normal cells have. They are dedicated to one function—reproduction. They are weak in the sense that a minor change in their environment may cause them to lose their reproductive function, and if that happens, the cancer stops growing. I believe that a radical change in diet, such as going on a macrobiotic diet, which is essentially grains and vegetables, can make a very significant change in our internal environment and make our cells inhospitable to cancer.

If you go the alternative route, how do you monitor your progress?

How do people know that alternative therapies are indeed working? They may perceive physical benefit, they may have less pain, they may have fewer symptoms. But does this really mean that the alternative therapy has had a significant effect? The way to monitor the success of an alternative therapy is to stay in touch with a traditional physician, to go back to that doctor and request the necessary tests to monitor the progress or the natural history of the disease. If the problem is a cancer of the lung, and after receiving or participating in an alternative therapy there is physical benefit and/or relief of symptoms, and a chest X ray does indeed show that the cancer is reduced in size, or is at least the same size, that would be a very good indication. The patient should be able to evaluate the effectiveness of alternative therapies, just as they should traditional therapies.

If you had only one message to give to cancer patients, what would it be?

Seek out the finest care available. Go to the physician most qualified to treat your illness. If that means traveling to a center in New York City that deals specifically with your type of cancer, that's what you should do. But you can't rest on that treatment. You can't be satisfied that you've done all that you can do. You must also will your way back to health. You must also participate in your own cure and be willing to meet the challenge of beating the disease. This means that you should participate in alternative therapies as well as traditional therapies. It means that you should not sit on the sofa and wonder if you are cured. Get up and run around the block and know that you are curing yourself. Participating in alternative cancer therapies in addition to traditional medical care will undoubtedly lengthen your life and improve your quality of life.

[All interviews have been edited for length and clarity.]

2

Dealing with Cancer

The Diagnosis

A diagnosis of cancer is devastating. It usually entails powerful feelings of fear, terror, and helplessness. It is a profound shock, often leading to disorientation and confusion. The overwhelming nature of these feelings can result in a variety of emotional responses, including depression, hopelessness, and denial.

The emotional shock is a natural response to frightening news. You should expect that you will be emotionally debilitated at first. Don't expect a lot of yourself; you will have some down time. Simply allowing yourself to experience the feelings is the most effective way through them, but this can take time and is not a skill all people have (see "Feelings" in chapter 7). This is the time to share your feelings and thoughts with family and friends. You can also, now or later, contact support organizations that will connect you with cancer survivors, or cancer patients who have recently been diagnosed (see Resources, section B). Talking helps reduce the intensity of overwhelming feelings and helps regain perspective and hope. Give serious consideration to seeing a professional counselor who is trained in helping people through an emotional crisis.

Remember, cancer is not the death sentence that it was once commonly believed to be. Some people survive virtually all forms of cancer, and there is no reason why you cannot be on the success side of your cancer's survival odds.

Gathering information can be very helpful. The more you know about your cancer, its treatments, and your choices, the more you reduce your fear of the unknown. Even simple efforts toward discovering answers to your questions can result in significant changes in the way you feel. By gathering information, you can replace the terror of helplessness with a sense that you have at least some control over the situation.

The sense of control or being empowered not only is useful in dealing with the cancer diagnosis, but is also an important element in maintaining hope and in surviving cancer. Loss of control leads to loss of hope, to depression and resignation. Having some sense of control means you can participate in and have some affect on the course of your illness. This can grow into a sense of power and to what is commonly called a "fighting spirit," which has been shown to increase the odds for survival.

Videotape

Cancer: Increasing Your Odds for Survival, narrated by Walter Cronkite. This is the four-hour public television series that is the companion to this book. The documentary was made to provide people with cancer with a resource for gathering information at a time when reading may be difficult due to the emotional shock of diagnosis. Available for $69.95 plus $5 shipping from:

New Way Productions
P.O. Box 8241
Manchester, CT 06040
phone: (888) 307-4482
Website: www.cancersurvival.com

Books

Neil Fiore, Ph.D., *The Road Back to Health: Coping with the Emotional Aspects of Cancer,* rev. ed. (Berkeley, CA: Celestial Arts, 1990). Fiore is a psychologist and cancer survivor, and he includes especially helpful sections on dealing with diagnosis and, as the title suggests, all the many emotional aspects of cancer.

Second Opinions

Second opinions are critical. Doctors and pathologists can make mistakes, and competency and accuracy differs from individual to individual and facility to facility. Of patients seeking second opinions at one major cancer center, 70 percent made changes in their treatment. Do not be afraid to ask to have your test results forwarded to another institution or doctor if necessary. Second opinions have become routine, and good doctors are not threatened by them.

Dr. Susan Love of the UCLA Breast Center recommends that you take the time, even with breast cancer, to get a second opinion. "A diagnosis of breast cancer is not an emergency," she says. "When diagnosed, you're so scared you'll do anything. It's important to let the shock wear off, get a second opinion, find out what is the best approach." Comprehensive Cancer Centers and other hospitals that specialize in cancer treatment are excellent sources for second opinions. A complete list of Comprehensive Cancer Centers can be found in Resources, section A. This and other information on hospitals that specialize in cancer care in your area is also available by calling the National Cancer Institute's Cancer Information Service at 1-800-4-CANCER (1-800-422-6237).

Multidisciplinary Second Opinions

At most institutions, cases are reviewed by an individual specialist at different times in the treatment process. Some institutions provide multidisciplinary second opinions. These are evaluations made by a panel of appropriate cancer specialists who meet together to review a case and share input at the same time. At institutions where this is offered, a patient can specifically request that such a team of cancer specialists review her or his diagnosis and treatment. Institutions that provide multidisciplinary second opinions are listed below. The R. A. Bloch Cancer Management Center in Kansas City, Missouri, maintains an up-to-date list of institutions providing these second opinions; phone 816-932-8453.

Little Rock, AR . . . St. Vincent Cancer Center 501-660-3900

Tucson, AZ . . . . . . Arizona Cancer Center 520-626-6044

San Diego, CA . . . University of California, San Diego,
                    Cancer Center 619-294-6394

San Francisco, CA . Regional California Foundation 415-775-9956

Denver, CO . . . . . . University of Colorado Cancer Center   303-315-3007

New Haven, CT . . Yale University 203-785-4175

Miami, FL . . . . Cedars Medical Center 305-325-4683

Atlanta, GA . . . . . DeKalb Medical Center 404-501-5559

Iowa City, IA . . . . University of Iowa Cancer Center 319-356-3584

Chicago, IL . . . . . . Loyola University Medical Center 708-216-9000

Baltimore, MD . . . John Hopkins Cancer Center 410-955-8964

Detroit, MI . . . . . . Karmanos Cancer Center 313-993-0335

Kansas City, MO . . R. A. Bloch Cancer Management
                   Center 816-932-8453

Lebanon, NH . . . . Norris Cotton Cancer Center 603-650-6300

Binghamton, NY . Regional Cancer Center Lourdes 607-798-5431

Bronx, NY . . . . Montefiore Medical Center 718-920-4826

Buffalo, NY . . . . . . Roswell Park 800-ROSWELL

New York, NY . . . . Ruttenbery Cancer Center 212-241-6470

Rochester, NY . . . . University of Rochester Cancer Center 716-275-4911

Cleveland, OH . . . Ireland Cancer Center 216-844-5432

Columbus, OH . . . James Cancer Hospital 614-293-8890

Philadelphia, PA . . Fox Chase Cancer Center 215-728-2986

Philadelphia, PA . . University of Pennsylvania Cancer
                   Center 215-662-4000

Providence, RI   . . . Roger Williams Cancer Center 401-456-2581

Knoxville, TN . . . . Thompson Cancer Survival Center . . . 423-541-1678

Memphis, TN . . . . St. Jude Children's (Children Only) . . 901-495-3306

Dallas, TX . . . . . . Arlington Cancer Center 817-261-4906

Galveston, TX . . . . UTMB Cancer Center 409-772-1164

Surgical Biopsy versus Needle Biopsy

Biopsies are procedures done to remove a sample of a tumor for testing to see if the growth is malignant, or cancerous. A surgical biopsy
uses surgery to open the patient; needle biopsies use a needle to
extract a sample. Inquire if a needle biopsy can be used for your
tumor. They are easier for the body to tolerate than a surgical procedure, and are about one-third as expensive.

Dealing with Doctors and Hospitals

Take the time to look for a doctor with whom you are comfortable. You do not have to accept the doctor assigned to you by the hospital. You may request another. Remember, you—or the insurance you paid for—are paying for your doctor.

Doctors are your consultants. Be sure your doctor agrees with your treatment philosophy. Good physicians should be open to new ideas and willing to help you in any way possible. This is especially important if you plan on using any leading-edge technology or complementary treatment. In our medical system, doctors need to order tests and procedures for you, you cannot order them yourself. Their willingness to request these tests will probably depend on their openness to new ideas and their dedication to your needs. Learn to ask for what you want. If you don't understand something, ask again. Write questions down, bring a friend or a family member to each consultation, and/or bring a tape recorder and tape your consultation if your doctor permits it. Be assertive. "Bad" patients survive longer.

The experience I had in the hospital trying to help Cindy was difficult, to say the least. We had tried to find a conventional doctor who would work with us, but once doctors learned that we were involved with an alternative treatment, they wanted nothing to do with us. Our reception at the local emergency room was similar.

I considered it my job to be Cindy's ombudsperson, her advocate. When we wanted to get a second opinion my task was to obtain a copy of her medical records and a CAT scan. Because Cindy had brain metastases that were considered untreatable in this country, she was labeled "terminal." We wanted to consult a German doctor who had successfully treated patients with cancer that had metastasized to the brain, but the hospital was not cooperative. In the conventional mindset, we were in denial and the hospital staff was working to protect us from quacks and charlatans by resisting providing medical records and test results. Although their assessment about denial may have been correct and their motivation altruistic, I do not believe they had the right to interfere with our obtaining help wherever we found a legitimate second opinion. We needed to feel that we had done everything within our ability to treat Cindy's illness, and their lack of cooperation interfered with this.

I sincerely hope you will not encounter resistance as we did, but you and your helpers should be ready. First, ask someone you trust who is hopefully skilled at dealing with people and bureaucracies to be your advocate in the hospital. This person can keep track of what is being done and help assure that what you need to have done is accomplished.

Consider requesting a copy of your medical records to have ready and on hand if you decide to change doctors or hospitals, or seek second opinions. As hard as it is to believe, access to your medical records can be legally denied in some states though most states in the U.S. provide for full disclosure to patients, and in most of the other states the hospital will provide records if requested to do so by your doctor. If you have difficulty with the hospital or your doctor, most hospitals have patient relations departments with staff who are there to help you.

Books

Lawrence LeShan, Ph.D., *Cancer as a Turning Point: A Handbook for People with Cancer, Their Families, and Health Professionals* (New York: Dutton/ Penguin, 1989). Includes an excellent chapter on dealing with hospitals, called "How to Survive in a Hospital."

Marion Morra and Eve Potts, *Choices: Realistic Alternatives in Cancer Treatment* (New York: Avon Books, 1980). Includes an excellent list of questions to ask your doctor.

Bernie S. Siegel, M.D., *Love, Medicine, & Miracles: Lessons Learned About Self-Healing from a Surgeon's Experience with Exceptional Patients* (New York: Harper & Row, 1986). Has a good section on "The Healing Partnership."

Booklets

Facing Forward: A Guide for Cancer Survivors includes questions to ask your doctor. It is available free by calling 1-800-4-CANCER.

Teamwork: The Cancer Patient's Guide to Talking with Your Doctor. Available free from the National Coalition for Cancer Survivorship; 301-650-8868.

National Cancer Institute (NCI)

The National Cancer Institute (NCI) is the federal government's primary agency dedicated to cancer research, diagnosis, treatment, and rehabilitation. It is responsible for disseminating information regarding these cancer topics, which it does primarily through the services listed below. It has designated over thirty comprehensive cancer centers with Cancer Information Services, which provide access to the database called Physician Data Query (PDQ, see below) and other cancer-related information, through the 1-800-4-CANCER number. It also offers cancer information through its Cancer Fax system, accessible via any fax machine, and through the Internet and libraries where cancer research and databases are available.

Access

Cancer Information Services Hotline: 1-800-4-CANCER (1-800-422-6237) for cancer-related questions

Cancer Fax: 301-402-5874
Call from a fax machine and request the Cancer Fax contents list.

NCI website: www.cancernet.nci.nih.gov
(Resources, section E offers a complete listing of cancer-related websites.)

Physician Data Query

The National Cancer Institute is aware that many patients are not receiving the most up-to-date treatments, usually because they are in smaller or rural hospitals with doctors who may not be aware of the latest cancer treatments. The Physician Data Query (PDQ) is one of the most important resources available through the Cancer Information Service of the National Cancer Institute. PDQ gives both patients and physicians information needed to help make appropriate decisions.

PDQ is a computer database containing treatment guidelines from the National Cancer Institute. It can help you determine if you are receiving the most up-to-date treatment. Treatment recommendations are given in two ways: the Health Professional file is written in language for doctors and other health care professionals; the Patient Information file contains similar treatment information but is written for the general public.

PDQ also contains a protocol file listing clinical trials that are accepting patients for experimental cancer treatments. The file can be searched by diagnosis and geographic location.

If you, a friend, or the local library have access to the Internet, PDQ's treatment recommendations and information on clinical trials can be found on the World Wide Web (www.cancernet.nci.nih.gov) and are also available by calling the Cancer Information Service at 1-800-4-CANCER. Treatment guidelines are also available from the National Cancer Institute's Cancer Fax service at 301-402-5874. You will receive easy-to-follow instructions about faxing treatment information for your cancer to you. All PDQ information is available at most medical libraries, although sometimes a fee is charged.

Support Groups

The importance of support groups cannot be overemphasized. Research indicates longer survival times for those participating in support groups. Besides potentially living longer, you can certainly live better with less stress by sharing your feelings and experiences with others as well as by learning from those who are going through a similar experience. Be aware that the quality of support groups, like the quality of doctors, varies widely. If you are in an area that has several, try different ones. Find a group in which you feel comfortable and where people share your intentions about doing whatever is necessary to survive cancer. Share your thoughts and feelings with your family and friends. Cancer is too big of an event to live through alone. Let others help.

See Resources, section B for a list of support groups.

Book

John Fink, *Third Opinion: An International Directory to Alternative Therapy Centers for the Treatment of Cancer and Other Degenerative Diseases* (Garden City Park, NY: Avery Publishing Group, 1997). Lists support groups and organizations.

Booklets

Facing Forward: A Guide for Cancer Survivors, When Someone in Your Family Has Cancer, and *Taking Time: Support for People with Cancer and the People Who Care About Them.* Excellent booklets available free from the National Cancer Institute. Call 1-800-4-CANCER.

Listen with Your Heart: Talking with the Cancer Patient. Available free from the American Cancer Society (ACS), 1-800-ACS-2345. Call ACS in the white pages to find out what support services are available from your local chapter.

Websites

Cancer Survivors OnLine lists hot lines:
www.ahamade.com/CancerSurvivors/

National Coalition for Cancer Survivorship:
www.cansearch.org/index.html

A Cancer Survivor's Story: Live the Pain, Learn the Hope:
www.dmgi.com/treelife.html

Cancer Care, Inc.: www.cancercareinc.org/

Children and Cancer

It was my original intent to include a section in the documentary with helpful information on childhood cancers. After interviewing Jeanne Munn Bracken, author of *Children With Cancer* (New York: Oxford University Press, 1986), I realized it was a topic deserving a documentary in itself. Not having any firsthand experience with a childhood cancer, I did not feel sufficiently knowledgeable to evaluate what was or was not helpful. The resources below will provide parents of children with cancer a starting point for their information needs.

Book

Jeanne Munn Bracken, *Children with Cancer: A Comprehensive Guide for Parents* (New York: Oxford University Press, 1986). Highly recommended.

Organizations

Candlelighters Childhood Cancer Foundation
7910 Woodmount Avenue, Suite 460

Bethesda, MD 20814-3015

Phone: 800-366-2223 or 301-657-8401

Provides information, support, and advocacy to families of children with cancer, survivors of childhood cancer, and professionals who work with them.

Websites

Children's Cancer Web Resources:

www.ncl.ac.uk/~nchwww/guides/guide2.htm

www.candlelighters.org

Insurance

Lack of health insurance, fear of losing coverage, and wondering if specific treatments are covered are stressful concerns for cancer patients. If you need to acquire insurance, look for a policy with the shortest exclusion for preexisting conditions. Also try to obtain a policy that guarantees you the right to renew, to avoid your insurance being canceled.

If you have insurance, be sure to send your payments on time to avoid giving insurance carriers any cause to cancel your policy. Keep accurate records of your bills and payments, and keep copies of any bills you submit to insurers.

Cancer survivor Anna Scala described some of her insurance concerns in her interview for the documentary *Cancer: Increasing Your Odds For Survival:*

> As a cancer patient, one of my biggest concerns was insurance. I had been paying for insurance for twenty-five years, and I never ever used it, never had a cold, never had anything. And when it came time for me to use it, they soon started increasing my monthly payments. So now they're close to $800 a month, up from $249 three years ago. And it's just been a daily battle with them, and there's no way I can change [insurance companies]. Every time I research it and talk to another insurance company, they ask, "Do you have an existing illness?" And as soon as you say yes, and then say what it is, they don't want you. Or the premiums are

so high you can't afford it. And you can't afford to be without it, either. I've gone as far as the insurance commissioner here in Connecticut, and he can't even seem to help. So I think [insurance is] one of the biggest concerns. People say, "Don't let it bother you," but it has to bother you. When you're facing a bill of $58,000, you can lose everything. You can lose your home, your business, everything. There's no way you can pay that.

Unfortunately, little can be done to prevent insurers from raising your rates. In cases of financial duress, some doctors and institutions try to help patients with their bills. If your plan covers 80 percent of the cost of treatment, ask the hospital or your physician to accept the 80 percent copayment from the insurer as a full payment.

If an insurance company refuses your claim, call the company and ask for an explanation. If their response is unclear or vague, ask to speak to a supervisor. If you believe your claim should be covered under your policy, ask about their appeals process, and write them a letter. As a last resort, you can talk to your state insurance commissioner's office or take legal action. This can be a frustrating and stressful area of concern that may require doing additional research and seeking increased support from friends, family, or patient advocates.

Book

Ralph Nader, William M. Shernoff, and Ruth Chew. *How to Make Insurance Companies Pay Your Claims, and What to Do If They Don't* (Mamaroneck, NY: Hastings House Publishers, 1990). If an insurance company rejects your claim, this book may be helpful in obtaining payment.

Booklets

What Cancer Survivors Need to Know About Health Insurance. Has an excellent Medicare summary. This and other resources are available at no cost from the National Coalition for Cancer Survivorship at 1010 Wayne Avenue, Fifth Floor, Silver Spring, MD 20910, phone: 301-650-8868.

Cancer Treatments Your Insurance Should Cover. Available free from the Association of Community Cancer Centers at 301-984-9496.

Facing Forward: A Guide for Cancer Survivors. Booklet that includes information on managing your insurance. Available free by calling 1-800-4-CANCER.

For Those with Limited Resources

If you do not have insurance, contact your local American Cancer Society, or call the Cancer Information Service at 1-800-4-CANCER, for information about community agencies that can assist in finding financial assistance for you. Your state Department of Public Health should also have information on community health clinics and public health programs.

Some hospitals and health care facilities, including nursing homes, have received federal assistance under the Hill-Burton program and are required to provide some free care. People with poverty-level income can apply for this assistance at participating hospitals. For a list of the health care facilities in your state, contact the following federal agency and leave a voice-mail message. To speak to someone about the program, call from 1:30 to 3:30 P.M. EST.

Organization

Office of Health Facilities
Health Resources and Services Administration
Department of Health and Human Services
5600 Fishers Lane, Room 11-03
Rockville, MD 20857
Phone: 800-638-0742

Bills and Viatical Settlements

Twenty percent copayments can add up fast. First, try to negotiate with the hospital or your health care provider. They will often settle for a reduced amount, especially if it means they will get something rather than nothing. Try to keep your credit intact. Paying a little of your bill each week will do that.

Hopefully it will not come to this, but there are companies that will purchase life insurance policies if you are terminally ill. These purchases are called "viatical settlements," and you can get between 50 and 80 percent of your policy's value. Settlements vary, so apply to more than one company. You might first check to see if your insurance policy has an "accelerated benefits" rider that will allow you to gain access to some of your insurance money before you die.

Booklets

Viatical Settlements: A Guide for People with Terminal Illnesses. Free from FTC Public Reference Branch, 6th Street and Pennsylvania Avenue, NW, Room 130, Washington, DC 20580.

What You Need to Know About Accelerated Benefits. Free from the National Insurance Consumer Hotline at 800-942-4242.

Trade Groups

Viatical Association of America, at 800-842-9811.

The National Viatical Association, at 800-741-9465.

Research Services

If you would like someone else to pull information on your cancer and treatment from the above sources, a research service developed by cancer survivor Gary Schine will provide a ninety- to three hundred-page report for approximately $200. Schine is the author with Ellen Berlinsky, Ph.D., of *Cancer Cure: The Complete Guide to Finding and Getting the Best Care There Is* (New York: Kensington Books, 1993). The service may be reached at

Schine On-Line Service
39 Brenton Avenue
Providence, RI 02906
Phone: 800-346-3287

Internet: Uses and Cautions

The Internet is an excellent resource for contacting people for information and support. It can be a good place to locate otherwise hard-to-find information, but be sure to carefully evaluate the source of whatever information you dig up. Medical libraries, hospitals, and level-headed researchers provide information—but so do unscrupulous vendors and well-meaning but misguided purveyors of inaccurate information. Use your judgment as to the reliability of your source, just as you would if the person were in the room talking with you. This is difficult when you have only written words from which to derive impressions. When information is critical, try talking on the phone with people to get a better sense of who they are and whether their information is valid. The Internet also can be useful for finding people who have had personal experience with various alternative and complementary therapies. If something has worked for others, it might work for you—but there is no guarantee. People have different cancers, and different bodies have different needs when it comes to cancer. If no one has had any success with a particular therapy, though, then it would seem logical to look elsewhere.

If you have no Internet experience, find someone to help you. If you are a new subscriber, start with a major service provider that has good customer support to guide you and includes established online cancer support groups. I recommend CompuServe because it seems to have better, more active cancer- and health-related groups, but look into all the major online services, including America Online and Prodigy. The quality of these online groups, just like support groups, can vary widely.

Book

Tom Ferguson and Edward J. Madara, *Health Online: How to Find Health Information, Support Groups, and Self-Help Communities in Cyberspace* (Reading, MA: Perseus Press, 1996).

Websites

See Resources, section E for a complete list of cancer-related websites.

Chapter Resources

Books

Marion Morra and Eve Potts, *Choices: Realistic Alternatives in Cancer Treatment* (New York: Avon Books, 1980). An excellent comprehensive guide to conventional treatment and issues. Highly recommended.

Richard A. Bloch, *Cancer... There's Hope* (Kansas City, MO: R. A. Bloch Cancer Foundation, 1981) and *Fighting Cancer: A Step-by-Step Guide to Helping Yourself Fight Cancer* (Kansas City, MO: R. A. Bloch Cancer Foundation, 1985). Bloch, of H & R Block, cured himself of terminal cancer. His books are available free by calling 1-800-4-CANCER. Both are excellent guides to a majority of major cancer topics and are inspirational and practical in their approach. Highly recommended.

Harold H. Benjamin, Ph.D., *The Wellness Community Guide to Fighting for Recovery from Cancer* (New York: Putnam, 1987).

Stephanie Matthews-Simonton, *The Healing Family: The Simonton Approach for Families Facing Illness* (New York: Bantam, 1984). Excellent, but out of print. Try your local used bookstore; many stores are hooked up to one another via computer to help find books.

National Coalition for Cancer Survivorship, *A Cancer Survivor's Almanac: Charting Your Journey,* ed. Barbara Hoffman, J.D. (Minneapolis, MN: Chronimed Publishing, 1996).

Support Groups and Organizations

Support groups and cancer-related organizations are listed in Resources, sections B and C.

Interview with Marion Morra

on Getting Information, Second Opinions, Family Issues, How Cancer Changes People, and Maintaining Hope

Marion Morra is a former assistant director of the Yale Comprehensive Cancer Center at Yale University School of Medicine, where she established the Cancer Information Service in 1975 and continued as project director until 1997. She is now an associate clinical professor at the Yale School of Nursing and president of Morra Communications, a firm that consults in health communications. She has written health- and cancer-related books and many articles. With her sister, Eve Potts, a medical writer, she wrote *Choices: Realistic Alternatives in Cancer Treatment*, one of the best compilations of cancer information I have ever come across; *Understanding Your Immune System; Triumph: Getting Back to Normal When You Have Cancer*; and, most recently, *The Prostate Cancer Answer Book: An Unbiased Guide to Treatment Choices*. She is a thoroughly dedicated professional who has always been willing to use her considerable knowledge and resources to help me locate hard-to-find information.

What is the first thing you suggest people do when they find out they have cancer?

Make sure that they know there is a lot of information [available] and that they find where to get that information. The 1-800-4-CAN-CER number is probably one of the main resources. Or, they can go to their local American Cancer Society office. Some people are information seekers, and they may end up going to medical libraries. And, of course, you need to ask a lot of questions from the health care providers, the doctors and the nurses who are going to be taking care of you.

Generally, what types of doctors and specialists will the cancer patient encounter?

Cancer patients will encounter several doctors along the way. Most cancer patients start with a surgeon because most have an operation: either a biopsy to make sure that [the tumor] is cancerous, or an operation to take the cancer out. They may or may not see a radiologist, who uses X rays for treating cancer. They may or may not see a medical oncologist, who uses drugs or chemotherapy for cancer treatment. They may see a social worker; they may see a dietitian. A lot of health professionals are involved in the cancer field, and it's really important for people to understand that those resources are there.

You said in your book Choices **that many people are not receiving the most appropriate treatment. Why is this, and how do you determine if your doctor is using the newest protocol?**

I think it's difficult for the general public to understand which is the newest treatment. It takes a long time for the newest therapies to get from the major centers in this country out into the general community. For example, we know that the children who come to the major treatment centers (with some types of childhood cancers) have an 87 percent cure rate. Yet, we know *overall* in the United States, for the same type of childhood cancer, the cure rate is probably down at 60 percent. And we know that it takes somewhere between five and fifteen years for the newest therapies to become standard practice in the communities. Now, for a cancer patient, that is a real dilemma. How do you know where and when you are getting the correct treatment?

One way to find out is to call the Cancer Information Service [1-800-4-CANCER] and ask them to do a PDQ search. *PDQ* stands for "physician data query," and it lists all of the protocols done in the United States that are listed on the National Cancer Institute databases. For over one hundred different kinds of cancers, you can have a search done that gives you the information on patients, the stages of the disease, and the kinds of treatments given. They will also do searches for a clinical trial for your stage of cancer in the area where you live, or anywhere else in the United States where the newest treatments are being given. Most of the newest treatments start at the Comprehensive Cancer Centers. These Comprehensive Cancer Centers are designated by the federal government—by the National Cancer Institute—as centers of excellence in cancer. They are scattered around the country, and that is where the newest clinical trials are being carried on. They go from there to the community.

Some hospitals and facilities specialize in a specific cancer. How do you find out about the capabilities of your hospital or doctor and therefore the best place for your cancer?

Yes, some places in this country specialize in one kind of cancer. There are also two or three hospitals in the United States that treat *only* cancer. You need to ask a lot of questions. You need to find out from your doctor how often he or she performs this specific operation. When you have one of the more common kinds of cancers, you will find, for example, that many of the community doctors can claim to do those operations several times a week. If you have an unusual kind of cancer, then it will be more difficult to find out where they do those operations often. I suggest that you go to a major medical center in that case. Unfortunately, people don't understand that. Nobody understands that there are doctors who only treat cancer of the uterus, who spend their entire lifetime doing that.

So, in those cases, it would be better to get your second opinion somewhere that might be farther away, and afterward ascertain whether your local facility is treating you with the latest protocol.

Yes, if the second opinion [from a major center] agrees with the first physician, you can decide whether to stay with the major center or go back to the local doctor. That is a personal decision people have to make for themselves. If the second opinion is the same as the first one and if the hospital you are at has good facilities, then there is reason to be treated by your local physician.

What are some of the most important things for parents of young children with cancer to be aware of?

Parents are real advocates for their children. They make sure that they get the latest in treatment; they make sure they ask all the difficult questions before the treatments are done. And most of the children with cancer are treated at major cancer centers. So their parents know, by the time the kids are treated, as much as the doctors know.

The parents and the kids form a team that is really important in the cancer treatment.

There are some problems that the parents face when they have a child with cancer, particularly when there are other children in the family. It's really hard on the other kids. Parents are worried about their child with the disease, and they spend a lot of time waiting in the hospital, bringing him to the doctor, caring for him—then the other kids act up. First of all, the siblings are frightened because their brother or sister has a disease. And second, they are sometimes jealous because of the amount of attention that the other child is getting.

However, there is a lot of help for these parents: wonderful, dedicated physicians and nurses; social workers; and people who work with the school system. We have a whole team of people who go out to the school system and help talk to the kid's classmates. There are many good resources in that area.

What are some of the normal problems associated with cancer and the family? What is your "checklist" for the family?

Family members are kind of forgotten in the whole area of cancer. When you are in the hospital, for example, the doctors visit early in the morning or late at night. And in the middle of the day, the surgeons are operating. So doctors visit at odd hours, when the family members are not present. But then, when the cancer patient goes home, the family has to take care of him or her. Thus, it's very difficult for the family members to get the amount of information they need to really understand what's happening, to be a part of the team that is taking care of the patient, to understand what the side effects are going to be, and to have a role in what happens to family members during that period of time.

There is a checklist in our book of what questions family members should ask and what kinds of things they should look at. How much do you talk to a cancer patient, and how honest can you be about your own feelings? Of course, if someone has a very serious diagnosis and the family member is afraid that the cancer patient is going to die, those conversations are really very hard.

Because so many people think that cancer is equated with death, we've also seen the other scenario: the family member prepares himself or herself for the patient to die, and the patient lives. There's a whole other set of problems—what do you do now that you have made all kinds of mental changes, thinking that the person was not going to live? There can be lots of resentment. So we try to tell people to be honest, to think about their own feelings, to do some normal things themselves. You can get caught up in trying to be the perfect person taking care of the cancer patient, and you forget that you need to have a life of your own. You need to get away. And you need to do those things without feeling that you are doing the wrong thing.

In *Triumph,* we have a whole section that looks at what kinds of things the family member can do for the patient and for themselves to make this time better. I think, also, that family members ought to understand that there are support systems for them out there. They can join support groups. They can see social workers at the hospital. Quite often people don't understand the role of the social workers— they are there to talk to people, to help them through their problems, to help with some of those communication issues. They are a very important part of the team of people who take care of cancer patients. At the hospital, I suggest that you ask for a consultation with the social worker because it will help family members sort through some of those issues.

Can you say something about the whole idea of a patient having advocates?

Family members can also be advocates for the cancer patients. We suggest that family members go with patients to the doctors' offices, and go with them when they are getting treated so that they can ask questions. Sometimes patients don't want to ask difficult questions because they want to have good relations with their health care team. But sometimes a family member can ask for them. For example, if the patient doesn't want to ask for a second opinion because he is afraid of hurting the doctor's feelings, the family member can say, "My brother really doesn't want to do that, but *I* want a second opinion for my own peace of mind." So there are things that family members can do as advocates when they are watching what happens.

It's really interesting to me that sometimes people seem to leave their sense of responsibility at home when they go to the hospital. You know, somebody gives you a green pill one day and a pink pill the next—don't you think you might ask, "Why did I get a pink pill instead of a green pill?" Mistakes are made: you might have gotten the medication that belongs to the person in the next bed. Somehow, people don't think that they should ask those kinds of questions. So I think that some family members can do that, but patients ought to be doing it themselves. You need to watch out for your own welfare.

What are some of the techniques once thought "way out" that are now being accepted by the mainstream providers?

There are all kinds of chemotherapeutic drugs that were used in only clinical trials but that are now standard treatment. Even some of the mental imagery and visualization techniques, when used in conjunction with the conventional treatments, are being looked at [more favorably]. Mental imagery and the connection between the mind and the body were explored before Christ. The Greeks looked at those issues. They aren't new. I think we are a long way from proving what it does because we don't know a lot about how the mind works. We are just beginning to explore those issues with the new technology. I think in the future we are going to see a lot of things in those areas that we don't know now.

What would you think about the idea that a person's psychology, their mental and emotional makeup, can have an effect on the outcome of the disease?

I think that when you have a serious disease, it's important to have a positive attitude. We know, for example, that information and hopefulness are connected. That's why I am big on saying you need to be part of the decision making; you need to go out and look for that information because that makes you more hopeful. That has been proven in some studies. And being more hopeful means having a positive attitude. It's saying, "I want to get to normal, I want to get back to work to make my life as good as it can be." It really doesn't matter how long you have to live. You really need to make sure that the days that you have are really good days. And that has to do with the kind of attitude that you have toward what happens. None of us know how long we have to live. It's just that the cancer patients must confront that. Most of us go through life thinking we are going to be here forever, and so you are never made to confront the possibility that you just might not have another hundred years.

Cancer patients, I think, are very different from the rest of us because no matter how long they live after they've had that diagnosis, they've confronted the fact that we are not immortal. I know a lot of cancer patients, and I know that they lead their lives very differently after they have gone through a cancer diagnosis. They are incredible people because they have done that. They really choose what they will do with the rest of their lives. I can't tell you how many cancer patients have said to me, "I don't have time to put up with all that nonsense anymore. I'm going to do what I want and need to do." I can tell you stories of cancer patients who had very little time left but who decided that the most important thing they needed to do was sail the Caribbean, and the physicians were able to allow them to do that. They got the chemotherapy down there. The rest of us don't live our lives in that manner.

A lot of cancer patients become much more impatient. They don't deal with nonsense anymore. They are in a hurry to get something done because it is important to them.

What are your suggestions for people to get their lives back together after the initial shock and after beginning treatment?

In doing *Choices* and *Triumph,* my sister and I talked to literally thousands of cancer patients. The material in the books is based on the questions people had: we asked people, as they were going through their experiences, to keep track of their questions and tell us, "What do you wish you had known? What were the surprises? What did you really want to know?"

It seems that the most difficult time for people was that between onset of some kind of symptom and the treatment. You are going through all those tests, you get the diagnosis, and you make a decision with the physician about treatment. That period of time is the hardest. Once you've made the decision and started the treatment, you get some control back in your life.

One of the things that helps you get that control is to get information and be part of the decision-making process. People feel, when they get a cancer diagnosis, that their body has done something terrible to them—particularly people who were feeling pretty healthy before they got it—it's not like you were feeling sick and then found out [the causes]. Most people have a vague symptom—they find a lump or see a spot—and they get a cancer diagnosis. They were going ahead thinking everything was all right and then learned something strange was happening inside them. And so I think that control issues for people are really important.

Most of the time when you are in a hospital, you don't feel like you are in very much control. Trying to be in control and trying to get back to some normal routine is very hard when you are undergoing cancer treatment, coming in every day for six weeks for radiation therapy. It is very hard to feel like you have control, and it is very hard for you to feel like you are living a normal life because, there is no doubt, you are not.

What we advise is to try to make other parts of your life as normal as you possibly can. If you used to like going to the movies or plays, try to see if you can make that a normal part of your life. Try to find a few things, here and there, that make you feel good. Take a little time off once in a while and go do something that is fun, instead of making a living out of being a cancer patient. We think you do better when you have some normalcy in your life.

If you had only one message to give cancer patients, what would it be?

Ask, ask, and ask again. You can never ask too many times. As a matter of fact, the doctors around here tell me that they know when patients have read our book because they come in with a list of questions. For most physicians—certainly for physicians who are in a medical center where students are always asking them questions—that's fine. They really like to feel that the patients are part of what is going on. When you see a cancer physician, it is not like seeing Marcus Welby, who knows everything that's going on in his patients' families. In real life, the cancer physician has probably never met you before and has absolutely no idea what is going on in your mind. So if you don't share some of [your experiences and concerns] and ask questions, he or she will never know the best types of treatments to recommend.

[All interviews have been edited for length and clarity.]

Marion Morra is president of Morra Communications, a health communications consulting firm, and can be reached there at 203-874-7923. Her books are available through bookstores and her website is www. cancer-books.com.

Part 2

Treatment

3

Conventional Treatment

There is no reliable, across-the-board cure for cancer. As some doctors have told me, conventional treatments cure a relatively small number of types of cancer. Few people argue about the value of surgery for removing tumors, especially if it is done early enough in the development of the cancer, as an effective treatment for localized cancers. The next step in conventional treatment is generally chemotherapy or radiation. Except for a few cancers, chemotherapy and radiation knock back the cancer, shrink tumors, may help control metastasis, and can facilitate at least a temporary, if not a complete, remission. However, they often fail to cure cancer. Because of their toxicity and potentially serious side effects, I suggest that you use chemotherapy and radiation, if they apply to your situation, carefully and with discrimination.

Some people forgo conventional treatment altogether. They pursue nontoxic alternative treatments, which if started early claim results similar to conventional medicine for some cancers. This is a risky road, especially with a fast-moving cancer. It is important to consider that one of the benefits of conventional treatment is that it can cause tumor regression and may even put the cancer in remission, buying you valuable time. This time can then be used for following up with other treatment modalities and complementary therapies such as psychotherapy (see chapter 7, "Psychological Aspects of Cancer").

Chemotherapy may also become less effective with each cycle, until it no longer has much or any effect. This is why doctors switch from one chemotherapeutic agent or drug to another, until there are no more chemotherapy drugs or combinations to offer.

Unfortunately, even the ability of chemotherapy to buy time is in question. Dr. Abel Ulrich, a respected cancer biostatistician and epidemiologist at the Heidelberg Tumor Center, published a controversial review of the literature on survival rates of patients with chemotherapy-treated cancer. He claims that chemotherapy alone can help only 3 percent of epithelial cancers (such as breast, lung, colon, and prostate), which account for about 80 percent of cancer deaths. As Ralph Moss, Ph.D., author of *Cancer Therapy: The Independent Consumer's Guide to Nontoxic Treatment and Prevention* (New York: Equinox Press, 1992) and *The Cancer Industry: The Classic Exposé on the Cancer Establishment* (New York: Equinox Press, 1996), advises in my documentary *Cancer: Increasing Your Odds for Survival,* you should always ask your physician for proof that the treatment you are being given will extend your life. This would seem to be good advice for any consumer, and especially so in situations where the treatment itself can be life threatening.

Book

Abel Ulrich, M.D., *Chemotherapy of Advanced Epithelial Cancer: A Critical Survey* (Stuttgart: Hippokrates Verlag, 1990).

Testing

Before you choose any treatment option, however, have tests done to determine the extent of your cancer so you have a baseline from which to start. Once done, these tests can be used to monitor the response of your cancer to the treatment or treatments you choose. Testing generally includes imaging, using technologies like X rays, ultrasound, magnetic resonance imaging (MRI), computed tomography (CT) scans, computerized axial tomography (CAT) scans, and nuclear scanning.

X-ray technology has progressed to the point where there is relatively little radiation exposure to the patient, as opposed to some of the other imaging methods. Many proponents of complementary medicine discourage the repeated use of X-ray and other imaging methods that require radiation to detect the presence or progress of cancer. There is debate over what if any negative effects this exposure has. If there are no other tests, my personal belief is that it is more important to know if the treatment is working than to avoid exposure to X rays.

Some tests, like CT scans, require greater radiation exposure, and questions regarding the effect of this exposure on DNA make this choice more difficult. MRI uses radiowaves and magnetic fields to produce highly detailed pictures with no known risk to the patient. Ultrasound uses high-frequency sound waves, which are also non-toxic, but the quality of the images and their usefulness depend greatly on the skill of the persons administering and interpreting the tests. All imaging methods require that the tumor be of a size that can be "seen" or measured by the technology.

There are blood tests that can detect the presence of some cancers in the body even if they are not detectable as a tumor mass. These tests have varying degrees of reliability, and include:

- the CA125 test for ovarian cancer,
- the PSA test for prostate cancer,
- CEA for colon, rectal, testicular, and breast cancer, and
- CA 15-3 for breast cancer.

Often, which tests doctors order are determined by what is available at their hospital. Ask your doctor, and your second-opinion physician, what the best tests for repeated evaluations of your treatment are, regardless of where they are available. Also remember to ask your doctors if they would be willing to continue to monitor your progress with testing if you decide to go the alternative or complementary route. I strongly recommend finding physicians who agree to this.

Testing: Anti-Malignin Antibody Screen (AMAS)

This new blood test for the existence or remission of cancer in a non-terminal patient is slowly gaining acceptance with some conventional doctors. *Nonterminal* means any patient whose cancer is not in the terminal phase of the disease. The test is called AMAS, and it examines the levels of anti-malignin antibody, which is elevated in malignancy and returns to normal values in cases of remission. The test is reported to be 90 to 95 percent accurate. Patients can use it as an indicator of whether or not a treatment is working, that is, whether the cancer is going into remission or is advancing or returning.

Many doctors are unaware of this test and may not be inclined to order it. It then becomes a challenge either to convince your doctor to order the test or to find a doctor or a walk-in health clinic that will. The test, and research information for your doctors' review, can be obtained from the following lab:

Laboratory

Oncolab
36 The Fenway
Boston, MA 02215
Phone: 800-922-8378

Testing: Tumor Aggressiveness

Routine analysis of a cancer tumor should be done to grade it. The grade of a tumor is usually associated with how malignant it is or how likely it is to spread or metastasize. This is often referred to as the *aggressiveness* of the tumor.

The two main types of aggressiveness testing or grading are *histological* and *nuclear.* Histological analysis is based on the **appearance** of the cells, or how similar the tumor cells are to normal cells. If the cancer cells have an orderly and distinct appearance similar to normal cells, they are said to be well differentiated and are a Grade One. Poor differentiation is an indication of a high-grade tumor. The grade is usually expressed in a range of either one to three or one to four, with one being a low grade with a lower chance of spreading, and the higher numbers representing a higher likelihood of the cancer's metastasizing.

Nuclear analysis is based on the **rate** at which cancer cells are dividing or proliferating and is done by a pathologist examining cell nuclei of the biopsy under a miscroscope. Nuclear analysis of the rate of tumor growth can include the measurement of *doubling time,* which is the average length of time it takes for the cancer cells in a tumor to divide and therefore double. Nuclear analysis of cell proliferation is expressed in a grade structure similar to histological analysis. Because these tests rely on the expertise of the pathologist, you may want to consider having your biopsy slides read by another pathologist at a different institution, like a Comprehensive Cancer Center (see Resources, section A).

S-phase fraction (SPF) testing measures the number of cells that are in their synthesis phase, or the phase at which they are ready to divide. It provides basically the same information as nuclear grading, but because it is done by computer it is generally considered more accurate. A high SPF may indicate that the tumor is more aggressive, but according to authors Steve Austin, N.D., and Cathy Hitchcock, M.S.W., in their book *Breast Cancer: What You Should Know (But May Not Be Told) About Prevention, Diagnosis, and Treatments* (Rocklin, CA: Prima Publishing, 1994), in some studies, a high SPF correlates with a worse prognosis, while in others it has made little or no difference.

Flow cytometry measures the "ploidy" status of the number of chromosomes in cancer cells. *Diploid* tumors have the normal number of chromosomes, are usually less aggressive, and are associated with a better prognosis. Tumors with an abnormal amount and type of DNA in the cell are called *aneuploid* and are usually more aggressive.

None of these tests is 100 percent predictive, and new tests are continually being developed, but taken together the results of existing tests can provide you with a probable assessment of how fast-moving or aggressive your cancer is. This can be valuable information in estimating the time you have to take action. Many—but not all—of these tests are routinely included in the pathology reports provided for your doctors at most hospitals. To be sure, ask your physician to request the tests that will provide you with the most information on tumor aggressiveness.

Testing: Chemosensitivity

A few hospitals now pretest chemotherapy agents against biopsy samples to determine which drugs are most effective against your particular cancer before you undergo a course of chemotherapy. Since cancers often develop resistance after the first round of chemotherapy, chemosensitivity testing is especially valuable in picking an effective second course of treatment. At one time, chemosensitivity testing was considered unreliable because it was only 50 percent accurate and it took too long to get the results. Today, preliminary results are complete in about nine days, and testing has progressed to the point where it is 85 to 90 percent accurate. This testing is not performed at all institutions, but it is available through a few specialized laboratories if you have your doctor request it.

In order to do this testing, a 200 milligram sample or biopsy of your tumor is necessary. If you are going to have a biopsy, request that enough tissue be gathered for this as well as for any other tests intended for the sample. You may have to overcome some resistance from doctors who are not aware of the current effectiveness of chemosensitivity testing and who may be reluctant to acquire a sample for this purpose alone. The following labs will provide you and your physician with in-depth information and research on the testing they provide.

Laboratories

Weisenthal Cancer Group
15140 Transistor Lane
Huntington Beach, CA 92649
Phone: 714-894-0011

Nu Oncology Lab
8052 El Rio
Houston, TX 77054
Phone: 713-747-6003

Surgery

In some cultures, folk wisdom maintains that surgery should be avoided if possible as it hastens the spread of cancer through the body. Maurice Finkel, M.S., Ed.D., is a practicing natural therapist in Australia, former president and cofounder of the Melbourne Chapter of the International Association of Cancer Victors and Friends, and a former professor of biology. In his book *Fresh Hope in Cancer: Natural*

Methods for Prevention, Treatment, and Control of Cancer (N. Devon, England: Health Science Press, 1998), he says there may be some scientific basis for this. Injuries or surgery stimulate the production of estrogen, which stimulates the production of repair cells as part of the healing process. This supposedly can stimulate the production of *all* cells, including cancer cells that may be located throughout the body but that might not yet be detectable. On the other hand, some research indicates that survival time doubles for those who receive surgery. This, in conjunction with many instances of people seemingly cured by surgery alone, would seem to make surgery a wise choice. However, using less invasive techniques like needle biopsies instead of surgical biopsies for testing, and lumpectomies instead of radical mastectomies (when possible), seems prudent in any case.

It is always important to be informed about the usefulness and type of surgery recommended to you. Taking the example mentioned above, lumpectomy (the removal of a breast cancer tumor and surrounding tissue) has been proven to be just as effective as radical mastectomy (removal of the entire breast) in many cases of breast cancer. Yet mastectomy is still performed in cases where it is not required. If your doctor recommends a mastectomy be sure there is a good reason for it, and obtain a second opinion.

Book

Richard A. Evans, M.D., *Making the Right Choice in Cancer Surgery: Treatment Options in Cancer Surgery* (Garden City Park, NY: Avery Publishing Group, 1995).

Timing of Breast Cancer Surgery for Premenopausal Women

According to the research of Dr. William Hrushesky at the Veterans Administration Medical Center in Albany, New York, breast cancer is less likely to metastasize fatally depending on when in the menstrual cycle breast cancer surgery is performed. The studies he cites indicate a two- to fourfold difference in ten-year survival, depending on when the surgery was done. According to Dr. Hrushesky, whom I interviewed for the documentary *Cancer: Increasing Your Odds for Survival,* immune function, as well as the potential to form new blood vessels necessary for cancer growth, changes during the menstrual cycle.

> If they [my patients] wish to time their surgery, I'll tell them, first of all, they have to be regularly cycling. And that they should plan to have the surgery between fourteen and twenty-three days after the first day of their last menstrual period. So, if their menstrual period begins today, they probably should wait somewhere around fourteen and sixteen days to have that surgery.

Similar timing might be important for these women to consider when scheduling biopsies. Although other researchers cite findings that challenge those of Dr. Hrushesky, he states that the majority of well-done studies confirm that there appears to be a benefit in timing the surgery close to ovulation and the week after. He also states that further studies are needed.

One argument used against timing breast cancer surgery to a woman's menstrual cycle is that this could cause unnecessary delay. This argument makes little sense, as it amounts to a delay of two to three weeks at the most, and may afford significant potential benefits.

Article

William J. M. Hrushesky, M.D., "Breast Cancer, Timing of Surgery, and the Menstrual Cycle: Call for Prospective Trial," *Journal of Women's Health* 5, no. 6 (Nov. 6, 1996): 555–66.

Organization

Dr. William Hrushesky, M.D.
VA Medical Center Oncology Department
113 Holland Avenue
Albany, NY 12208
Phone: 518-462-3311 ext. 2792
Website: rpi.edu/~hrushw

Circadian Timing of Chemotherapy Delivery

The time of day a chemotherapeutic drug is given also has an impact on the effectiveness of the drug, its toxicity, and how much damage is caused to the immune system and other cells in the body. Delivery at optimal times in the day increases quality of life for patients by decreasing the toxicity they experience, and it also allows physicians to increase the average dose that can be given.

Unfortunately, most hospitals are not set up to see patients at multiple times during the day. Some hospitals, however, are beginning to take advantage of a variety of drug delivery devices, such as drug infusion pumps, which are capable of administering chemotherapy (and other drugs) at different times and different rates throughout the day. These devices can be plugged into a subcutaneous catheter access port, which is commonly used for delivering chemotherapy, and chemotherapy can then be administered at the optimal times.

Ask your doctor or find a hospital capable or willing to set you up with a programmable drug infusion pump for your chemotherapy.

Optimal times for delivery of many common chemotherapy drugs are known and published; see the chapter below in the medical textbook edited by DeVita, Hellman, and Rosenberg.

Books

William J. M. Hrushesky, M.D., ed., *Circadian Cancer Therapy* (Boca Raton, FL: CRC Press, 1994).

Vincent T. DeVita, Jr., M.D., Samuel Hellman, M.D., and Steven A. Rosenberg, M.D., Ph.D., eds., *Cancer: Principles and Practice of Oncology* (Philadelphia: Lippincott, 1992). See article on pp. 2666–86, "The Application of Circadian Chronobiology to Cancer Treatment."

Radioactive Seed Implants

Radioactive seed implants are small radioactive pellets that are placed near a cancer tumor to deliver a highly localized form of radiation therapy. This treatment is becoming available for many forms of cancer and is less toxic and damaging than many other forms of radiation. It is not available in all hospitals, so ask your doctor or call the National Cancer Institute's information line (1-800-4-CANCER) to find out if and where it is available for your type of cancer.

Hormonal Therapies

Breast, prostate, colon, and ovarian cancers are considered to be hormone related. Hormonal, or endocrine, therapy changes the hormonal balance in the body to make it less conducive to cancer cell growth. Since estrogen can promote the growth of cancer cells, the original endocrine therapy consisted of surgically removing the ovaries in premenopausal woman, and this can still be effective in cases of metastatic breast cancer.

Today, a variety of hormonal agents are used, including lupron, megace, and aminoglutethimide. First, estrogen receptor tests are done to ascertain if the patient's cancer cells are sensitive to hormones and will therefore be responsive to hormonal therapy. Tamoxifen is another drug that can help block the effect of estrogen. However, the effects of tamoxifen in the body are complicated, as is the understanding of when they are best used and on whom. This is another reason why a second opinion at a major cancer center is a good idea: it can help assure you that you are being offered the most current and safe treatment choices. Hormonal therapies are, in some cases, as effective as chemotherapy and deserve your attention as a treatment option, if they are available for your cancer. In many cases it is recommended that they be tried even *before* chemotherapy.

While hormonal therapies do have side effects, a major advantage is that they are usually less toxic than chemotherapy. You should discuss these side effects—which include nausea, vomiting, fluid retention, weight gain, possible infertility, and changes in sexual desire—with your doctor.

Dr. Susan Love is a respected breast surgeon who has worked at the Dana Farber Cancer Center in Boston and who cofounded the National Breast Cancer Coalition. She is a proponent of many innovative approaches to cancer treatment. In *Dr. Susan Love's Breast Book* (2d ed., Reading, MA: Addison-Wesley, 1995) she says:

> Most medical oncologists are better trained in giving chemotherapy than endocrine [hormonal] therapy, and they derive a greater profit from it as well. It just may not occur to them to try a hormonal maneuver first unless you bring it up. Certainly the best quality of life is likely to be associated with the less toxic but successful hormonal treatments.

Books

Susan M. Love, M.D., with Karen Lindsey, *Dr. Susan Love's Breast Book*, 2d ed. (Reading, MA: Addison-Wesley, 1995). Contains detailed information on hormonal treatment for breast cancer.

Steve Austin, N.D., and Cathy Hitchcock, M.S.W., *Breast Cancer: What You Should Know (But May Not Be Told) About Prevention, Diagnosis, and Treatments* (Rocklin, CA: Prima Publishing, 1994). Contains excellent summary of the pros and cons of tamoxifen.

Dealing with the Side Effects of Chemotherapy

Nausea

Today there are a variety of conventional antinausea drugs that your doctor can prescribe to control the nausea that is one of the most uncomfortable side effects of chemotherapy and hormonal therapies.

Relaxation, biofeedback, self-hypnosis, and imagery techniques are often used by patients and increasingly are offered at hospitals to help patients deal with nausea. If your clinic does not offer any and you are interested, resources for meditation and imagery found in chapter 6 of this guide are a good starting point.

Some herbal remedies can also help. These include: chewing on a slice of fresh ginger; drinking a heaping teaspoon of arrowroot mixed with six ounces of water; and drinking peppermint, licorice, chamomile, or ginger herbal teas.

Hair Loss

Ask your doctor about an "ice cap," or cold cap, that can be worn during chemotherapy. The cold restricts the flow of chemotherapy to the hair follicle, thus avoiding or reducing hair loss in some cases.

Radiation Burns

According to Stephen Fulder, in his book *How to Survive Medical*

Treatment: A Holistic Guide to Avoiding the Risks and Side Effects of Conventional Medicine (Woodstock, NY: Beekman Publishers, 1995), vitamin E applied to the treatment area before and after radiation treatment can prevent burning and diminish subsequent pain and scarring. He also recommends applying aloe vera gel to burns to assist healing and avoid scarring.

Reducing Toxicity and Damage to Immune System

Eating a diet high in calories, proteins, and vitamins can help prevent some of the damaging effects of treatment and rebuild the body's immune system and strength.

According to Stephen Fulder, the herbs *Astragulus, Ligusticum,* and *Codonopsis* are effective in restoring immune function, but he recommends taking them under the advice or care of a professional herbalist or acupuncturist.

In some studies, vitamin E increased the effectiveness of some chemotherapies and radiation and reduced the toxicity of some chemotherapies.

In other studies vitamin C increased the effectiveness of radiation, decreased side effects, and helped protect bone marrow. It may reduce the ability of the blood to clot and so should probably be avoided before surgery.

Coenzyme Q10, or CoQ10, is an antioxidant that has also been shown to prevent cell damage from chemotherapy.

Books

Stephen Fulder, *How to Survive Medical Treatment: A Holistic Guide to Avoiding the Risks and Side Effects of Conventional Medicine* (Woodstock, NY: Beekman Publishers, 1995).

W. John Diamond, M.D., and W. Lee Cowden, M.D., with Burton Goldberg, *An Alternative Medicine Definitive Guide to Cancer* (Tiburon, CA: Future Medicine Publishing, 1997). Contains information on complementary medicine useful to counter side effects.

Marion Morra and Eve Potts, *Choices: Realistic Alternatives in Cancer Treatment* (New York: Avon Books, 1980). Contains suggestions regarding the effects of treatment and diet.

Booklets

Eating Hints: Recipes and Tips for Better Nutrition During Cancer Treatment, Radiation Therapy and You: A Guide to Selp-Help During the Treatment, and *Chemotherapy and You: A Guide to Self-Help During the Treatment.* Guides to self-help during treatment. All are free from 1-800-4-CANCER.

New Generation of Conventional Cancer Treatments

Advances in understanding the genetics and biology of cancer are beginning to lead to the development of a new class of effective treatments, including biologic response modifiers, immunotherapies, monoclonal antibodies, vaccines, and gene therapies.

Biologic response modifiers (BRMs) are substances that alter the response of specific elements of the immune system to enhance, restore, or direct the immune defenses of the body. By definition, biologic response modifiers include several fields of research, including immunotherapies, vaccines, and immune-enhancing agents. These types of therapies are often referred to as *biologic therapies.* (They are not the same as the biologic therapies of complementary medicine, which are similar in intent yet are achieved usually through nutritional approaches.)

One BRM therapy is interferon, a protein molecule manufactured by the body that helps combat certain diseases, including cancer. Synthetic interferon is being used to treat a number of cancers. Although interferon usually does not cure cancer, it usually helps control some cancers, and it increases survival times.

Immunotherapy tries to engage a patient's immune system in fighting cancer. Recombinant interleukin-2, or IL-2, was developed by Dr. Steven Rosenberg and his colleagues at the National Cancer Institute. It is the first immunotherapy approved for clinical use that uses the patient's own immune cells to fight cancer. IL-2 consists of killer cells taken from a patient, coded to attack cancer, and grown to large numbers with interferon.

Vaccines are another promising form of therapy being developed. As with many of this new generation of experimental treatments, vaccines are difficult to classify because cross-fertilization of technology has inspired researchers to create approaches using immunological, biologic, and genetic sciences. Several vaccine approaches are being explored. One uses specific markers, or antigens, present in the surface of cancer cells to help the patient's cancer-fighting T cells locate and destroy them. This approach was used for a vaccine that resulted in significant shrinkage of melanoma tumors for 47 percent of patients involved, and it offers real hope for less toxic treatments for other cancers as well.

Other promising discoveries involve telomerase, an enzyme that causes cancer cells not to age and die like normal cells. Researchers hope that inhibiting this enzyme will cause cancer cells to die and that this will lead to a treatment for many, if not most, forms of cancer. Another encouraging development is the discovery of the p53 gene, which is responsible for stopping 60 percent of cancers from growing. Researchers at the M. D. Anderson Clinic in Houston, Texas, inserted the p53 gene into an inactivated cold virus and injected the virus with the p53 gene in it into lung tumors. In four of six advanced lung cancer patients, cancer tumor growth was stopped.

Gene research has resulted in the development of a new treatment for breast cancer. Researchers have discovered the gene responsible for the overproduction of the protein HER-2/neu, which drives the growth of malignant cells in 25 to 30 percent of breast cancers. This has led to the development of Herception, an antibody that counteracts the protein and can slow or stop some breast cancers from growing.

New therapies are slowly becoming available, and many more are being tested in clinical trials (see "Clinical Trials," below). Because developments in this group of new treatments are rapid, people must rely on their doctors and on sources like the Physician Data Query (see "Physician Data Query," chapter 2) to be sure they are not missing a more effective treatment opportunity for their cancer. Unfortunately, you cannot always rely on your doctor to be aware of these developments, especially if you are in smaller or rural hospitals. At a lecture on immunological cancer treatments I recently attended, a man in the audience had not been told at his hospital that interferon was an option for his melanoma. To be sure that you are informed of the latest treatments for your cancer, either get a second opinion from a major medical cancer center, such as a Comprehensive Cancer Center (see Resources, section A), or consult the Physician Data Query.

Photodynamic Therapy (PDT)

Photodynamic therapy, also called "phototherapy," uses a light-absorbing chemical that accumulates in abnormal cells. When the drug is exposed to light in the form of a laser, cancer cells are destroyed and normal tissues spared. This form of therapy has shown some very promising results in some hard-to-treat cancers. In Japan, it has been used for some lung cancers with phenomenal results. If treatment with or clinical trials of this therapy are available for your cancer, they merit serious consideration.

Angiogenesis

Angiogenesis is the formation of small blood vessels within the body, which is necessary for cancer tumor growth. Many researchers are looking for ways to cut off the blood supply to tumors to stop their growth. The alternative treatment of shark cartilage is claimed to be effective because of its ability to inhibit angiogenesis (see "Shark and Bovine Cartilage" in chapter 5).

One of the most promising developments in cancer treatment is the combining of the drugs angiostatin and endostatin. These are proteins that have been remarkably effective at preventing and destroying small blood vessels, or preventing their formation, around tumors in mice. There is great hope that this process may result in a treatment that can stop virtually all forms of cancer from growing. Clinical trials offering this treatment deserve your serious consideration, but trial size is very limited compared to the number of people interested. Many similar therapies are being tested in other trials, including AE-941, an extract of shark cartilage. Be aware that some agents that prohibit angiogenesis in mice have not worked in humans.

Articles

Judah Folkman, "Fighting Cancer by Attacking Its Blood Supply," *Scientific American* 275, no. 3 (Sept. 1996): 150–54.

J. Folkman, T. Boehm, T. Browder, and M. S. O'Reilly, "Anti-angiogenic Therapy of Experimental Cancer Does Not Induce Acquired Drug Resistance," *Nature* 390 (Nov. 27, 1997): 404–7.

Clinical Trials

Clinical trials are experimental programs in which cancer patients are offered new treatments or new combinations of established treatments. Clinical trials are often the last line of defense for conventional medicine in cases where no other treatment has worked. Clinical trials usually test new conventional medicines, but recently, through the efforts of the Office of Alternative Medicine, more research is also being done on alternative treatments.

In order to establish a baseline for comparison, research studies are often conducted so that participants will not know if they are in the treatment group or the control group, which is the group receiving no treatment. If this is the case for the clinical trial you are interested in, be sure that the possibility of being in the control group is acceptable to you. Preliminary research is usually available. Ask your doctors for information on the success of treatments being tested and on possible side effects, if known. Besides determining curative effect, clinical trials try to identify side effects and set the appropriate therapeutic dose. Be aware that in some cases side effects may be serious and that as an experimental therapy it may or may not work. Many new therapies are emerging, and your doctor should be aware of the clinical trials available for your cancer; if not, contact 1-800-4-CANCER, or consult the Physician Data Query.

Noteworthy Conventional Treatment Centers

There are many excellent hospitals specializing in cancer treatment. For the Comprehensive Cancer Centers nearest you, and for other hospitals and clinics that specialize in treating your specific cancer, call 1-800-4-CANCER. (See Resources, section A for a list of Comprehensive Cancer Centers.) Some other significant cancer treatment centers are mentioned below.

Cancer Treatment Centers of America

The Cancer Treatment Centers of America is an association of three hospitals, one in Zion, Illinois, another in Tulsa, Oklahoma, and a third in Portsmouth, Virginia. Their holistic approach combines conventional treatment with some progressive complementary therapies. They can be reached at 1-800-FOR-HELP.

Robert Janker Clinic

This cancer clinic is run by Wolfgang Scheef, M.D., who uses a variety of immune stimulants and chemotherapies, including one chemotherapy drug virtually unavailable in the United States. Dr. Scheef uses aggressive short-term chemotherapy because he believes this causes less damage to the immune system and bone marrow than does the standard low-dose, long-term chemotherapy used in the United States. Because of the intense chemotherapy he uses, he requires that a person's liver be no more then 50 percent affected by cancer.

Robert Janker Clinics
Baumschulallee 12–14
53115 Bonn
Germany
Phone: 011-49-228-7291-0

Chapter Resources

Research

The National Cancer Institute (NCI) provides access to PDQ and other cancer-related information through its Cancer Information Services hot line, 1-800-4-CANCER. It also offers cancer information through its Cancer Fax system, accessible via any fax machine, and through the Internet and libraries where cancer research and databases are available.

Cancer Information Service hot line: 1-800-4-CANCER for cancer-related questions
Cancer Fax hot line: 301-402-5874
Website: www.cancernet.nci.nih.gov

Consulting Service

Cancer Consulting Group (CCG) is a group of doctors and scientists that provides specific cancer information to patients, relatives, physi-

cians, hospitals, and corporations. They provide one-on-one consultation, by phone or e-mail, with cancer specialists who will empower
you to deal most effectively with any problem or issue related to your
cancer. Their clients have used CCG to gain access to the most
sophisticated standard or experimental therapies and to investigate
the research data on alternative therapies ranging from gene therapy
to green tea. They also have represented patients to their insurance
companies or HMOs regarding reimbursement for bone marrow transplants, have encouraged primary care physicians to make appropriate
referrals, and have documented the value of procedures for physicians
who are denied payment. Their clients include cancer centers, drug
companies, hospitals, corporations, and individuals. There is no charge
for an initial consultation.

R. Michael Williams, M.D., Ph.D.
P.O. Box 802
Island Lake, IL 60042
Phone: 847-526-8692
E-mail: through website: www.nulab.net/ctn/

Books

Marion Morra and Eve Potts, *Choices: Realistic Alternatives in Cancer
Treatment* (New York: Avon Books, 1980). This is a must-have book, excellent on conventional treatment, and open-minded and intelligent.

National Coalition for Cancer Survivorship, *A Cancer Survivor's Almanac:
Charting Your Journey,* ed. Barbara Hoffman, J.D. (Minneapolis, MN:
Chronimed Publishing, 1996).

Booklets

*Fact Book: National Cancer Institute, Chemotherapy and You: A Guide to Selp-
Help During the Treatment, Radiation Therapy and You: A Guide to Selp-Help
During the Treatment,* and *What Are Clinical Trials All About?* Free booklets
available from the National Cancer Institute. For copies of these and other
booklets, call 1-800-4-CANCER.

Interview with
Bruce Chabner, M.D.

on the Availability of State-of-the-Art Treatment, Special Considerations for Older People, Being an Informed Consumer, Key Points for Survival, and Testing Unconventional Treatments

Bruce Chabner is the chief of Medical Hematology and Oncology and the director of the Clinical Cancer Center at Massachusetts General Hospital. He was the director of the Cancer Treatment Division at the National Cancer Institute from 1982 to 1995.

The National Cancer Institute campus in Bethesda, Maryland, with its many research institutions and divisions, is an impressive collection of resources and individuals dedicated to finding a cure for cancer. No less impressive is the obvious dedication of Dr. Bruce Chabner, who directed its treatment division for many years.

What is the first thing people should do when they find out they have cancer?

Get the best possible opinions about the seriousness of the situation and about how it should be treated. That includes having the pathology reviewed to be sure that it *is* cancer and to be sure that you know what kind of cancer it is, and then asking for an expert opinion about how to treat it. Often the diagnoses are made at a community hospital by people who are not very familiar with management of cancer, and so people in that situation need to go to a cancer center, or at least to a physician who is an expert in dealing with that particular kind of cancer.

Many people are not receiving the most appropriate treatment. Why is that?

We aren't sure how many people are receiving appropriate treatment and how many people are not. First of all, in some instances, it's hard to define what is appropriate treatment. But in other instances—for example, in the management of certain forms of early breast cancer—we know what is appropriate treatment, yet there are significant numbers of patients who still don't get it.

The reasons are that the practice of medicine changes slowly, that surgeons who are used to doing mastectomies don't like to do lumpectomies. Or radiation therapy, which is an alternative to radical surgery for breast cancer, may not be available in all communities for a number of reasons. It takes time to change patterns of practice and to reeducate physicians. There are also probably some economic incentives for maintaining certain outmoded practices. People don't like to give up patients; they don't like to refer patients to cancer centers because it's a loss for their own practice. I think as physicians become better educated, and as the new crop of physicians who *are* educated about dealing with cancer go into practice, things will change for the better.

I read somewhere that older people are more likely not to receive state-of-the-art treatment. Why is that?

Yes. Older people are a problem for treating cancer because often they can't tolerate the same kind of treatment that would be given to a younger patient—more radical kind of surgery or chemotherapy or very intensive radiation therapy. Both patient tolerance and the quality of life that will result from the treatment are important factors in deciding treatment.

There's also a tendency, I think, for physicians to underestimate what an older patient can tolerate. And they often make decisions just on the basis of [the patient's numeric] age without considering what we call the "physiologic age," the fitness level of a patient. Some older people in their sixties or even seventies are very fit and able to go through regular kinds of treatment, chemotherapy, radical surgery. So mistakes are made sometimes in that regard.

There are some studies showing that older patients don't handle drugs as well. They don't get rid of them as quickly, and [they accumulate] more toxicity, so there is, certainly, an additional risk of treating an older patient—with chemotherapy in particular. But by and large, most patients can be managed through this and can tolerate therapy when it's necessary and important.

What is the potential benefit of all people receiving state-of-the-art, or appropriate, treatment?

We think, from just looking at the cancer statistics, that bringing state-of-the-art care to all patients might be significantly beneficial. For example, if you look at the statistics about diseases like non-Hodgkin's lymphoma, you see that death rates are actually not going down as we would expect, knowing what we can do for those patients. And we suspect the reason is that many of these patients are not receiving state-of-the-art care. A look at the national cancer statistics for specific diseases that we know are treatable gives us the impression that we could do better.

So, basically, the major potential benefit would be saving lives?

Yes, I think that, sure. And we could avoid all the problems of inappropriate treatment. If you don't get the right treatment in the beginning, then you have lots of complications later on: hospitalizations, treatments that don't work, pain and suffering, and having to live with cancer. So it's better to get the right treatment right up front, even though it may be more expensive and inconvenient, and also probably more toxic initially. But if it cures you, you're much better off.

How do you determine if your doctor is using the newest protocol, and if you think he or she is not, what should you do?

It's difficult to determine whether your doctor is using the best protocol. Probably the easiest way is to go to a recognized center for treatment of cancer. Usually the doctors that are practicing there are involved in the very latest protocols and the testing of new drugs. There are also many very fine private practices of medical oncology, for example, or surgery, where the doctors participate in clinical trials. Ask the doctor that you're going to, "Do you participate in clinical trials (or studies)?" Usually, doctors that do that are aware of what is the best and state-of-the-art.

Board certification is also important. Now there are specialty boards—examinations given to qualify doctors to practice cancer specialties—particularly in medical oncology and radiotherapy. If you are receiving drugs from a medical oncologist, he or she should be board certified, as should a radiation therapist.

What do you think is the most important thing for a cancer patient to be doing to survive?

Be a well-informed consumer—know what's being done to you and why. Get the best possible care; go to the best possible physician, even if it's inconvenient. Follow your doctor's instructions; don't try to make changes in midstream. Ask for second opinions when a problem arises or if a serious decision must be made. I guess, overall though, the most important thing is to find the right doctor and the right institution. That's the decision you make initially, and that's the one that's really crucial.

What did you think of the OTA [Office of Technology Assessment] report on unconventional cancer treatments? Was it balanced?

I think it was reasonably balanced, although I think that some of its conclusions weren't entirely fair. They felt that there wasn't an avenue for testing unconventional agents. In fact, we have tested some unconventional drugs in the past, such as hydrazine sulfate and laetrile. We're willing to test things that we don't even understand, things that don't have a great scientific rationale, if there is any reasonable evidence that they work. We've never been opposed to testing the unconventional on the grounds that they were proposed by unconventional people.

We *do* have a standard, though. There has to be some reason to test it, some evidence that it works. Let me also add that it's possible, if one went to an extreme, for either consumers or scientists to waste a lot of good money chasing after unconventional therapies. I think we have to prioritize things by how good they are scientifically.

What is your opinion on psychoneuroimmunology? Do you think the psyche can affect the immune system, and could its effects potentially make people's immune systems less capable of dealing with carcinogens?

There's no doubt that there are connections between the brain and the immune system; they share a lot of the same receptors and proteins involved in transmitting messages. We don't fully understand how it works. I think there probably are instances in which people's attitudes affect how well they deal with cancer and whether they in fact get a malignancy. I can't cite any great evidence for this. It's a very difficult field to work in. But most of us are convinced that there are important connections between the brain and the immune system.

Do you think approaches like meditation, relaxation, and imagery as supplemental treatments are worth it for people to look into?

I really don't know. I don't think there's much hard evidence to prove that imagery and other psychological techniques are important in cancer treatment or survival. We do think that it's very important for patients to have strong support from family and from support groups of other patients and to have a positive attitude. The cancer patient has to go through a lot. There's a lot of mental anguish associated with hearing that diagnosis and taking the treatment. It's easy for patients to give up and to become very discouraged.

I'm not sure that a positive attitude influences the outcome [survival rate], but it certainly can influence how well a [family copes]. Does the family remain intact? Does that person deal with it and come out a pretty wholesome individual, or is the person scarred for life by the experience? All those things are affected by the patient's attitude.

You were talking about support systems earlier: which supplemental therapies would you say are useful?

I think maintaining a good lifestyle with a lot of exercise. A balanced diet is important. Putting some enjoyment in your life so that you're not obsessing about the diagnosis and the treatment. It's like any other crisis in a person's life—marital crises, or crises with your children or other things. The more support you have and the more wholesome you are as a person going into it, the better you are going to deal with it. A lot of families and a lot of marriages just have a hard time coping with it.

If you had one message to give to cancer patients, what would it be?

I think the single most important thing for a patient who has just found out they have cancer is to be sure they are at the best possible institution. It could be a private practitioner, or it could be a cancer center or a local hospital; but one has to be sure that that hospital or that practitioner can offer the very best.

How do you tell that? Well, cancer centers are the best guarantee. But also, you can tell by the degrees, the fact that your doctor is a specialist in this area and has a lot of experience dealing with it. And you will have to trust your sense of the doctor's competence, and whether they are able to tell you exactly what's going on, and whether you trust what they say.

[All interviews have been edited for length and clarity.]

4

Alternative Treatments

Conventional treatments are better for some cancers than others. If conventional treatment offers little or no hope of a cure, alternative therapies can represent continued hope in the quest for survival. The terms alternative and unconventional treatments generally refer to therapies that are not approved of by mainstream medicine. These therapies may also be called nontoxic, holistic, and complementary, and names that connote a negative value like questionable, unproven, and unorthodox. Although "alternative" does at times refer to a treatment that is used instead of a conventional treatment, it can also refer to a complementary or supplemental approach, which is a therapy used in *addition* to the conventional treatment. Supplemental therapies are like adjuvant or adjunct therapies in conventional medicine: they are used to complement a primary therapy by decreasing side effects or by enhancing the effects of the conventional treatment to help avoid reoccurrence of the cancer. Therapies discussed here have been used both as alternatives and as supplements to conventional medicine.

Alternative therapies are validated by varying degrees of research and often are supported by only limited research and anecdotal evidence. They are not approved by conventional medicine. Why, then, are more people searching for alternative treatments? In 1990 a report from the Office of Technology Assessment, *Unconventional Cancer Treatments* (Washington, DC: GPO, Report OTA-H-405), found that "effective treatments are lacking for many cancers, especially in advanced stages; many mainstream treatments entail considerable toxicity; and long-term survival may be uncertain even after apparently successful treatment."

Alternatives have not been successful for all people all of the time, but they have worked for some people. As I said before, when the odds are extremely low with conventional treatment, alternatives may offer the only hope.

Advocates estimate that overall alternative treatments have helped cure about 10 percent of the people who have used them. This is obviously a very general figure, but if you consider it a cure rate, it is certainly better than zero. So, should everyone try alternatives? No. Ten percent odds are not great. But if your chances are 0, 1, or 2 percent, then 10 percent is better, and your odds can probably be increased by careful research and homework.

Despite some improvement in research and testing in recent years, alternative treatments are still a gamble. The field of alternative medicine lacks consistency. Critics say alternative treatments are costly and are little more than fraudulent quackery. Although some unscrupulous alternative practitioners undoubtedly exist, many individuals and doctors base their commitment to alternative treatments on the success they have had treating cancers considered untreatable by conventional methods.

Many alternative treatments work to improve the person's natural immunity to fight the disease. One of the drawbacks of conventional treatments is that chemotherapy and radiation reduce immune system function. Some alternative approaches maintain that their immune-enhancing therapies will work better if the patient's immune system is not damaged by chemotherapy and radiation. However, in many cases cancer tumors are effective at avoiding immune response. Proponents of natural approaches believe this can be changed if the body is returned to a natural, balanced energy state, and some alternative treatments or regimens are directed at achieving this.

Choosing an Alternative Treatment

What a body needs to foster healing differs from individual to individual. Only research and self-awareness can determine which approach and which treatment, if any, is right for you. If you plan on pursuing an alternative or complementary course of therapy, I recommend that you consider using a research service and obtain the books listed at the end of chapter 5; these books will provide further information and resources.

The first step in choosing an alternative treatment is knowing your odds with conventional treatment. This can tell you how seriously you need to consider an alternative approach, and give some indications of the issues that may be critical for you. No matter what your odds are, complementary therapies should be able to increase your survival odds and improve your quality of life. As with any treatment, however, do not rush to action before you have done your homework.

As I said earlier, some alternatives work for some people and not for others. This may be due to the different types and potential causes of cancer. What one person's body needs to correct an imbalance or to fight cancer may be completely different from what someone else needs. The challenge is to find the treatment that is right for you.

Plenty of information can be found on alternative treatments, but there is no repository of independent, unbiased evaluations. This is what advocates for the Office of Alternative Medicine at the National Institute for Health had hoped for, but only limited information on alternative approaches is available so far (see "Organizations," below). Some alternative providers simply do not have the resources to follow up and compile data on their patients and treatments. Others inflate their success rates, or approach evaluations with an inherent bias. Be skeptical while keeping an open mind.

If you can afford to, enlist the aid of a research service familiar with alternative treatments, such as People Against Cancer or Ralph Moss's service (see "Research Services," below). They are familiar with the success rates of various alternative treatments as they apply to specific types of cancer. This knowledge is crucial and is time consuming to research. A good research service can narrow your search to the therapies most effective for your specific cancer.

A laboratory that will test your biopsied tumor against a variety of alternative medicines could provide you with most helpful information. Unfortunately, I know of only one such lab at this time (see "Pretesting Therapeutic Agents for Your Specific Cancer," this chapter). Laboratory tests can provide the most direct indication of the potential some alternative approaches may have for your cancer.

If you are unable to afford these options, you must rely on your research skills and those of your helpers. A good starting point is this guide. The alternative and complementary approaches mentioned in this book are the ones that I believe, after eight years of studying and exploring the field, offer the best chance of increasing survival odds.

Once you identify a therapy that you are interested in, ask the alternative treatment provider which cancers respond best to that treatment. Ask about the response rate of your type of cancer to the treatment, and request documentation on the therapy success. When a response rate is given, make sure you understand their definition of *response*. For some, a response may mean short-term improvement, for others, a remission or cure. Ask the practitioner for names and numbers of others who have used the therapy. If providers do not comply with your request, you should be wary. Call other patients and ask about the pros and cons of the treatment, what they know about other people using the therapy, and if it works for them. Look for support groups that might supply names of people who have tried various alternative treatments and who are willing to talk about their experiences. Internet newsgroups are another way to find people who have tried alternative approaches, but if you are not already familiar with the Internet, taking the time to learn may be frustrating.

Here is a starter list of questions to ask yourself as you consider an alternative therapy or approach:

- Do you believe in the approach?

- Does it match or conflict with your belief system?

- Do you have the time to do what is required?

- Can you afford it?

- Are you physically capable of doing what is required?

- Does the therapy require a level of financial commitment that you are unable or unwilling to make?

- Does the therapy require a level of time commitment that you are unable or unwilling to make?

- Does the therapy require a level of support from family or friends that you are unable or unwilling to obtain or accept?

The process of choosing an alternative program is generally more intuitive than scientific. There are no guarantees, but you can help stack the odds in your favor by considering the questions above. Once you have decided on a course of treatment, *make sure you have access to testing to determine if the treatment is working* (see "Testing Treatment Progress," below). Find out from the provider the average time in which results occur with the therapy. If testing indicates the therapy is not working, be prepared to try something else. If at all possible, use testing from unbiased, external sources, and do not rely on the provider's testing. If the provider discourages testing, find another therapy.

If you are thinking of using an alternative as a supplemental or "adjuvant" therapy, be sure to ask the alternative provider and your conventional doctor if there are any known compatibility problems. Some vitamins may reduce the effectiveness of some chemotherapies. Some alternative treatments don't work well with other alternative approaches. Because so many substances and potential combinations have yet to be tried, very few of these interactions are known.

Most of all, don't lose hope. If you begin to get overwhelmed, step back and talk to family, friends, and professionals. Take the time to regroup, gather your information in small pieces, and enlist the aid of others. Once you have decided on a course of action, stick to it until it is time to test, and be ready with an alternate plan that, hopefully, you will never have to use.

Books

John Fink, *Third Opinion: An International Directory to Alternative Therapy Centers for the Treatment of Cancer and other Degenerative Diseases* (Garden City Park, NY: Avery Publishing Group, 1997). Includes a directory of alternative practitioners with provider information of types of cancer treated. Also contains support groups and a good chapter on guidelines for choosing a therapy.

Ralph W. Moss, Ph.D., *Cancer Therapy: The Independent Consumer's Guide to Nontoxic Treatment and Prevention* (New York: Equinox Press, 1992).

Richard Walters, *Options: The Alternative Cancer Therapy Book* (Garden City Park, NY: Avery Publishing Group, 1993). Has good suggestions for choosing a therapy.

Organizations

The organizations below can provice patients with contacts for alternative therapies.

International Association of Cancer Victors and Friends
7740 W. Manchester Ave., Suite 110
Playa del Rey, CA 90293
310-822-5032

Cancer Control Society
2043 North Berendo St.
Los Angeles, CA 90027
(213) 663-7801

Research Services

The Health Resource
564 Locust Street
Conway, AR 72032
Phone: 501-329-5272

Operated by cancer survivor Janet Guthrie, the Health Resource provides an excellent comprehensive report on the latest conventional, complementary, and alternative treatments for your cancer and stage. Clients receive an in-depth research report that contains: information on conventional and alternative treatments for their specific cancer; a computer search of the medical literature on their cancer; a list of relevant clinical trials; copies of the latest medical journal articles discussing treatments for their cancer type; information on coping with chemotherapy and radiation therapy (herbal, nutritional, and psychological techniques); suggestions for immunostimulation; and a list of recommended books on cancer. Bound reports are 110 to 150 pages in length and cost $350 plus shipping. Clients not satisfied with the report can return it within thirty days for a full refund. Health Resource researches both mainstream and complementary therapies and does not advocate any specific type of therapy. It is a highly knowledgeable resource for people with cancer.

The Moss Report
144 St. John's Place
Brooklyn, NY 11217
Phone: 718-636-4433

A cancer report service operated by Ralph Moss, Ph.D., author of *Cancer Therapy: The Independent Consumer's Guide to Nontoxic Treatment and Prevention* (New York: Equinox Press, 1992). Ralph Moss is a critical thinker and is especially knowledgeable about alternative treatments. He will provide you with a forty- to fifty-page report containing "detailed and prioritized information on practitioners and treatments that he feels are the most valid and relevant to your situation." The cost is $275.

People Against Cancer
Alternative Therapy Program
P.O. Box 10
Otho, IA 50569-0010
Phone: 515-972-4444

A nonprofit membership organization that provides counseling and educational materials on nontoxic, innovative forms of cancer prevention, diagnosis, and therapy. They have a unique Alternative Therapy Program, available to people who join People Against Cancer as sustaining members for $350. Members provide a medical history and records, blood tests, and liver profile. Information is faxed to appropriate selected physicians, who report how successful their therapy is with that specific cancer and stage. People Against Cancer is not affiliated with any physician or clinic but acts as an advocate for its members by providing unbiased information.

World Research Foundation
41 Bell Rock Plaza, Suite C
Sedona, AZ 86351
Phone: 520-284-3300 or 818-999-5483 (in CA)
Fax: 520-284-3530

A nonprofit service organization that gathers, stores, and distributes medical information from ancient healing practices to modern conventional and alternative treatments. The foundation offers two different types of information packages, one dealing with the latest allopathic (conventional) medicine, and the other a library search of complementary and nontraditional approaches. This is an excellent potpourri of articles and research at a very reasonable price: library searches cost around $70.

Pretesting Therapeutic Agents for Your Specific Cancer

Before undergoing a complete course of therapy, you may want to take advantage of the tests that are available to determine which substances are most effective against your cancer (see "Testing: Chemosensitivity" in chapter 3).

The laboratory listed below will test your cancer against a variety of alternative treatments and may be able to test against specific alternative and complementary therapies.

Laboratory

Rational Therapeutics
Cancer Evaluation Center
3601 Elm Avenue
Long Beach, CA 90807
Phone: 562-989-6455
Website: www.rational-t.com

For testing, obtain a biopsy of your cancer tissue. You must not have received chemotherapy or radiation in the past four weeks. The cost is $2,000 to $2,500. Insurance coverage depends on your policy.

Testing Treatment Progress

It is imperative that you have access to diagnostic testing to evaluate the success of the alternative treatment you choose. You need to work with or have access to an open-minded doctor who is willing to order follow-up tests.

Testing can be as simple as ultrasound for some tumors, and cancer markers for others. Conventional science excels at this (see "Testing" sections in chapter 3 for an overview of available tests). Beware of tests used by the provider of an alternative treatment. Ideally, you want independent testing. Before treatment, you want to have established a baseline that determines the status of your cancer. You then can have the test redone after a course of treatment to see if the alternative is working. Ask your doctor, and your second-opinion physician, what the best tests are for repeated evaluations of your treatment.

Office of Alternative Medicine

The Office of Alternative Medicine (OAM) was established in 1992 as a division of the National Institutes of Health (NIH). The congressional mandate establishing the OAM stated that the office's purpose is to "facilitate the evaluation of alternative medical treatment modalities" to determine their effectiveness.

The OAM's first year was devoted to identifying the alternative medicine community and identifying barriers to the evaluation of complementary and alternative medical practices.

In June 1992, an ad hoc advisory panel was convened to address these two major objectives.

The group issued a report, published in December 1994, about the status of complementary and alternative medicine in the United States, *Alternative Medicine: Expanding Medical Horizons* (Washington, DC: GPO, Stock no. 017-040-00537-7).

The OAM looks at alternative medicine as it relates to all diseases, not just cancer. The OAM has funded ten Specialty Research Centers to study complementary and alternative treatments for specific health conditions. The University of Texas Health Science Center, in Houston, houses the center that specializes in cancer, and it has an excellent website.

At the present time, the results of a few OAM-funded research projects using alternative approaches to cancer are available only on the OAM website. They hope to have hard copies of their research results available soon through their toll-free clearinghouse number.

Other than reporting on its own research, the OAM does not offer any evaluative information on alternative treatments. General information about OAM and a list of OAM-sponsored research projects are available by calling the clearinghouse or through their fax-back system.

Report

Office of Alternative Medicine, *Alternative Medicine: Expanding Medical Horizons* (Washington, DC: Government Printing Office, 1994). This 428-page report costs $25 and is available from:

Government Printing Office
Superintendent of Documents
P.O. Box 371954

Pittsburgh, PA 15250-7954.
Phone: 202-512-1800
Fax: 202-512-2250
GPO stock number: 017-040-00537-7

Organization

OAM Clearinghouse
P.O. Box 8218
Silver Spring, MD 20907
Phone: 888-644-6226
Fax-back System: 800-531-1794
Fax: 301-495-4957

Websites

Office of Alternative Medicine: altmed.od.nih.gov. Choose "Research Grants," then "Grants Award and Research Data," then "OAM Grants Database"; then type in the search word *cancer.*

University of Texas Center for Alternative Medicine, Houston: www.sph.uth.tmc.edu/utcam/

Specific Alternative Treatments

Remember, alternative treatments are sometimes difficult and demanding regimens. They require personal motivation, dedication, and faith. They are not necessarily exclusive of other treatments, and most but not all usually can be used as complementary therapies. Below are a few of what I believe are the most promising alternative and complementary therapies out there.

714-X

Scientist Gaston Naessens, at the Cose Institute in Rock Forest, Quebec, has developed a powerful microscope that makes it possible to observe living blood at magnifications previously not possible. Using this microscope, Naessens has identified previously unseen particles, which he has named "somatides," and has observed that they have a degenerative cycle.

People with cancer have fewer somatides than normal, and degenerated forms of somatides are present in those with advanced cancer. By observing the condition and number of somatides, Naessens is able to predict cancer in individuals. Using this technology, he has developed 714-X, a natural, supplemental treatment that is meant to restore the blood and immune system of people with cancer.

Former Iowa Congressman Berkley Bedell, who was the founding force behind the creation of the Office of Alternative Medicine, believes it was 714-X that allowed him to survive prostate cancer. Canadian authorities brought Naessens to trial in an attempt to stop him from distributing an unapproved therapy, but so many people testified to its effectiveness that he has been allowed to continue his work in Canada. (You can read *The Galileo of the Microscope: The Life and Trials of Gaston Naessens*, by Christopher Bird [see below], for the complete story.)

Presently, the FDA has issued an "import alert" on 714-X, making it illegal to bring it into this country. When I asked an FDA official why 714-X, which I have heard good things about, had an import alert, I was told that the FDA had received information from a Canadian government agency, "National Health and Welfare Canada," that alerted them to 714-X.

The FDA official sounded sincere in his belief that the FDA was involved in protecting the American people from an unscrupulous product. However, he and I differed in our belief that governments are always indisputably reliable and accurate sources of information.

Gaston Naessens was tried unsuccessfully in Canadian courts twice. If 714-X was not outlawed by Canadian courts and is available in Canada, it is hard to understand why it is outlawed here. The product is inexpensive, but United States citizens must travel to Canada and receive treatment there.

Book

Christopher Bird, *The Galileo of the Microscope: The Life and Trials of Gaston Naessens* (St. Lambert, Quebec: Les Presses de l'Université de la Personne, 1990).

Organization

CERBE Distribution, Inc.
Center for Somatidian Orthobiology

5270 Rue Fountaine
Rock Forest, Quebec, J1N3B6, Canada
Phone: 819-564-7883
Fax: 819-564-4668
Website: www.cerbe.com

Burzynski Antineoplastons

The controversial Dr. Stanislav Burzynski of the Burzynski Clinic in Houston, Texas, has been researching peptides that regulate cell growth within the body and that form a natural defense against cancer. Peptides, which are protein fragments, are found in the blood and urine of healthy individuals but are generally lacking in the blood of people who have cancer. Dr. Burzynski's treatment consists of giving cancer patients these peptide combinations, which he calls "antineoplastons."

In October of 1991, The National Cancer Institute sent a team to look at Dr. Burzynski's cases and concluded that he had indeed caused a remission, either complete or partial, in seven cases of brain cancer that had been untreatable by all other means. According to Ralph Moss, Ph.D., author of *Cancer Therapy: The Independent Consumer's Guide to Nontoxic Treatment and Prevention* (New York: Equinox Press, 1992), in his interview for the documentary *Cancer: Increasing Your Odds for Survival,* Dr. Nicholas Patronas, M.D., Chief of Diagnostic Radiology at the Clinical Center at the National Institutes of Health, who was part of a team sent to evaluate Burzynski's work, observed that in the twenty years he had been in the business, Burzynski's were the best results he had ever seen. The treatment is supposed to work best on brain, prostate, and bladder cancers and lymphomas. Treatment is expensive, and insurance coverage might be difficult to obtain.

Ironically, the state of Texas has been trying to shut down Burzynski's clinic for many years. As of this writing, Burzynski has been cleared of all legal actions.

Book

Thomas D. Elias, *The Burzynski Breakthrough: The Century's Most Promising Cancer Treatment . . . and the Government's Campaign to Squelch It* (Los Angeles, CA: General Publishing Group, 1997).

Institute

Burzynski Research Institute
Outpatient Clinic
1200 Richmond Avenue, Suite 260
Houston, TX 77082
Phone: 281-531-6464

Energy Medicine

Energy medicine is a new term being used to describe a range of old and new medical and therapeutic applications of therapies ranging from the electrical to the spiritual. It includes therapies that use the more scientific or tangible energies, such as electrical, magnetic, electromagnetic, and electrochemical energies, and therapies that use the more subtle human body energy referred to in Eastern traditions as *chi, ki, prana,* and *etheric energy.* Energy medicine includes therapies such as acupuncture and chi-kung, disciplines born of the Eastern medical view that the body is an energy system and that disease results from blockages in the natural flow of energy (see "Acupuncture" and "Chi-kung," chapter 5).

It is a fact that the body has an electromagnetic field: the research of Dr. Harold Saxton Burr of Yale University in the first half of this century found that indications of disease were apparent in the body's electrical field long before physical symptoms emerged. Dr. Joseph Issels, a German pioneer in the use of a variety of alternative and complementary therapies, maintained that a change in the body's polarity protected tumors from attack by the immune system, and he used magnetic fields to alter the polarity, thereby allowing the immune system to attack the cancer.

In the 1930s, Raymond Royal Rife, an American inventor of medical technology working at his research laboratory in Point Loma, California, was reported to have used electrical frequencies to kill cancer cells as he viewed them through a powerful microscope of his invention. Since that time, many people are experimenting with frequency generators. Ideally they are used in conjunction with microscopes (such as dark-field microscopes, which are specially adapted to project high magnification and contrast images on a video screen) capable of observing their effects, since some frequencies may actually stimulate cancer growth.

This work has been taken in a similar direction by Dr. Bjorn Nordenstrom, former head of diagnostic radiology at the Karolinska Institute in Stockholm, Sweden, and chair of the Nobel Prize Assembly. Nordenstrom discovered electrical polarities in the bloodstream and has been able to manipulate the electrical currents within some untreatable tumors with successful results.

Another electrochemical cancer therapy showed promise in a research project sponsored by the Office of Alternative Medicine (OAM) at the City of Hope National Medical Center in Los Angeles, California, under the direction of Chung-Kwang Chou, Ph.D. As stated on the website of the Office of Alternative Medicine,

> In a preliminary study, treating mouse and rat fibrosarcomas with proper levels of direct current, inserting both anodes and cathodes into the base of tumors, resulted in long-term tumor-free animal survival . . . . These animal studies are significant since rat fibrosarcoma is very difficult to cure; radiation, chemotherapy, and even surgery are ineffective. More rigorous engineering and biological studies, both in vitro and in vivo, must be conducted to provide a solid foundation for this promising, simple and economical alternative method for treating localized tumors.

Electrical cancer therapies are considered experimental and are largely unavailable in the United States.

Books

Robert Becker, M.D., *Cross Currents: The Promise of Electromedicine, The Perils of Electropollution* (Los Angeles, CA: J. P. Tarcher, 1990). Represents the classic publication in the field. Not cancer specific.

John Fink, *Third Opinion: An International Directory to Alternative Therapy Centers for the Treatment of Cancer and Other Degenerative Diseases* (Garden City Park, NY: Avery Publishing Group, 1997).

Article

Bjorn Nordenstrom, M.D., "Electrochemical Treatment of Cancer, I: Variable Response to Anodic and Cathodic Fields," *American Journal of Clinical Oncology* 12 (1989): 530–36.

Website

Office of Alternative Medicine: altmed.od.nih.gov. Choose "Research Grants," then "Grants Award and Research Data," then "OAM Grants Database." At the keyword search prompt, type *cancer*

Organization

International Society for the Study of Subtle Energy Medicine
356 Goldco Circle
Golden, CO 80403
Phone: 303-425-4625

Practitioners

Various practitioners using therapies of the type pioneered by Rife and Nordenstrom can be found in John Fink's book, *Third Opinion* (see above).

Entelev and Cancell

Entelev was developed by James Sheridan, a chemist and cancer researcher from Michigan, with a degree from Carnegie Institute of Technology, who researched an approach to the chemistry of cancer that came to him in a dream. His Entelev formula includes inositol, potassium, sodium, copper, and bioflavonoids and was designed to work on the electrical aspects of cells. The Humanitarian Organization of People for Entelev (HOPE, not to be confused with HOPE Cancer Health Society), a support group for Entelev and cancer patients, estimates that the substance is approximately 80 percent effective against most cancers, and there are countless anecdotal stories of terminal patients being cured.

Unfortunately, we might never fully understand the benefits of this promising compound, since it came under suspicion from established medicine early in its development. Sheridan distributed the formula free of charge to cancer patients until 1983, when a court injunction prevented him from doing so. From 1984 to 1992, Edward Sopcak, a chemical metallurgist, took up the cause and distributed Entelev free of charge using the name Cancell. After eight years, he changed the formula to more of a homeopathic type of solution that he believed imparted a beneficial "vibrational" effect, although at first he continued to call his formula Cancell. At this point, Cancell received some media attention and was largely discredited because of its less definable and more questionable nature. Sopcak eventually changed the name of his formula to Quantrol, but not until the damage to Cancell's reputation had been done. Sopcak, like Sheridan, was taken to court by the FDA and was ordered to stop giving away his formula, although proponents of this formula also claimed it to be effective. Sopcak's formula is the focus of the book *The CanCell Controversy,* by Louise Trull (Norfolk, VA: Hampton Roads, 1993), which also contains documentation of Sheridan's theory, research, and efforts at obtaining FDA approval for Entelev.

The original Entelev formula is available from Medical Research Products in Miami under the name of Cantron. It is offered as part of an overall wellness program with no claims as to its effectiveness for cancer or other diseases. It costs $170 for a six-month supply. Proponents claim that if it is effective at all, the results will be evident in one to three months.

Organization

Ollie Blezinski, contact person
Humanitarian Organization of People for Entelev (HOPE)
27640 Van Horn
New Boston, MI 48164
Phone: 313-783-5558

Website

www.best.com/~handpen/Cancell/cancell.htm

Source

Medical Research Products
3960 NW 167th Street
Miami, FL 33054
Phone: 800-443-3030 (within the U.S.); 305-628-9981 (outside the U.S.)

Gerson Therapy

Gerson therapy is a classic diet and detoxification program consisting of organic juices and vegetables, coffee enemas, and enzymes available at the Gerson Institute in Tijuana, Mexico (619-585-7600). The city of Tijuana has become synonymous with the many unapproved therapies and, in some cases, unscrupulous clinics established there to avoid FDA regulation. This tainted reputation is unfortunate in the case of Gerson therapy, which by many accounts is worthy of investigation. Dr. Max B. Gerson (1881–1959) was a German physician, about whom the famous physician Albert Schweitzer once said, "I see in Max Gerson one of the most eminent geniuses in medical history."

Gerson therapy was a mainstay of the treatment at the Centro Hospitalario Internacional Pacifico, S.A. (CHIPSA), in Tijuana, until new developments in cancer treatment resulted in the establishment of the Gerson Research Organization. The Gerson Institute split off and continues to offer the classic Gerson treatment. The Gerson Research Organization continues to work at CHIPSA and offers an impressive variety of promising, well-known alternative treatments, including Coley's toxins and Dr. Joseph Issels's autogenous vaccines.

Organization

The Gerson Research Organization
7807 Artesian Road
San Diego, CA 92127
Phone: 800-759-2966 (within the U.S.); 800-754-0466 (from Canada)

Govallo's Immunoembryotherapy

Valentine Govallo, M.D., Ph.D., director of the Moscow Medical Institute's Laboratory of Clinical Immunology (CITO), has developed an anticancer vaccine derived from cells obtained from human placentas. For sixteen years, he has treated patients diagnosed as incurable, and he claims that more than 70 percent have survived over ten years with tumors either reversed or halted.

Organization

People Against Cancer
604 East Street
P.O. Box 10
Otho, IA 50569-0010
Phone: 515-972-4444
Website: www.dodgenet.com/nocancer

Iscador

Iscador is a derivative of mistletoe and has long been used as a cancer treatment in Europe. Iscador is administered either as a single agent after surgery, or as part of a broader treatment enhancing the immune system. Clinical studies in Germany, Switzerland, India, and Norway have shown Iscador effective in destroying cancer cells, preventing recurrences, and prolonging survival rates in solid cancers (cancers of the "solid" organs, like brain, lung, liver, colon, breast, and prostate, as opposed to cancers of bone marrow or lymph nodes). Unfortunately, Iscador is not an approved drug in this country. As such it is available only through doctors who are willing to acquire it from the manufacturer in Germany using the appropriate legal process, "eIND" or "compassionate use" law, or by writing letters on behalf of patients, who can then acquire it under the "personal importation policy." (See "Compassionate Use: Acquiring Unapproved Therapies," below.) A homeopathic form (*viscum compositum*) is available through Biologic Homeopathic Industries in New Mexico, which also provides numbers for mail-order suppliers.

Suppliers

Weleda (U.S. distributor)
175 North Route 9W
Congers, NY 10920
Phone: 800-241-1030 or 914-268-8574

Biological Homeopathic Industries
P.O. Box 11280
Albuquerque, NM 87123
Phone: 505-293-3843

Organization

Association for Anthroposophical Medicine
1923 Geddes Avenue.
Ann Arbor, MI 48104
Phone: 313-930-9462
Fax: 734-662-1727

Clinic

Lukas Klinik
CH-4144 Arlesheim
Switzerland
011-41-61-72-3333

The Kelly/Gonzalez Program

Donald William Kelly was a dentist who became interested in the German physician Max Wolf's work with enzymes and who developed his own cancer therapy. Kelly believed that certain enzymes were responsible for controlling cancer and were missing in those with cancer. His work has led to a variety of Kelly program derivatives. Besides providing enzymes, Kelly's program consists of diet, supplements, juicing, and detoxification techniques, including coffee enemas. Dr. Nicholas Gonzalez, in New York City, is one of the better-known practitioners of the Kelly program. This is the alternative therapy that Cindy chose after discovering that her breast cancer had metastasized.

Gonzalez prefers patients whose immune systems have not been compromised by chemotherapy and radiation, since these patients have greater success with his program. He believes that his program is the only one that works and that dedication and commitment to his treatment approach are essential for survival.

Although the program is demanding, Cindy was willing to put forth the effort if it meant she would live. Our principal problem with the program, however, was the lack of testing and supervision. Dr. Gonzalez did not use X rays, believing that they contributed to cancer, and he discouraged frequent progress checks, saying that "pulse takers" did not do well on the program. Given the lack of monitoring of the disease progress, I cannot recommend Gonzalez's program to those interested in the Kelly therapy.

Some people interested in the Kelly approach have followed a metabolic program (see "Diet: Metabolic Programs" in chapter 5) of nutrition and detoxification, adding the enzymes to it and being monitored closely by a physician to evaluate if the enzymes were working.

Dr. Jack Taylor, an Illinois chiropractor and licensed nutritional counselor, is a good source of nutritional information regarding the

Kelly program and metabolic typing. Pancreatic enzymes and other high-quality vitamins and supplements are available from Nutri-Supplies, below.

Practitioner

Jack Taylor, M.S.F., D.C.
3601 Algonquin Road, Suite 801
Rolling Meadows, IL 60008
Phone: 847-222-1192

Supplier

Nutri-Supplies
2695 North Military Trail, Suite 7
West Palm Beach, FL 33409
Phone: 800-388-8808

Livingston Cancer Treatment Program

The Livingston program was developed by Virginia Livingston, M.D., and consists of dietary changes, supplements, immune system stimulants, cleansing techniques, and vaccines. Livingston claimed she discovered a microbe that caused cancer, and she developed a vaccine that was reported to be very successful at treating cancer. I mention Livingston's program because it is my understanding that the original vaccine formula is no longer offered, for legal reasons. The therapy as it is offered now is a comprehensive dietary and nutritional program that may still be useful as a complementary therapy.

A study published in the *New England Journal of Medicine* followed a group of patients who had cancers for which conventional treatment was effective only 20 percent of the time (or less). Patients receiving orthodox treatment were compared to those treated with the Livingston program; it was found that both were equally ineffective at extending life. This seems to indicate that diet alone is not a sufficient or reliable treatment for cancer, and especially not at the terminal stage. It also raises the question of why people with similar diagnoses and stage three cancers are still treated with chemotherapy if this study showed that it did not extend life. Interestingly, the study also indicated that patients found the quality of life to be better with conventional treatment than with the Livingston program, indicating that alternative treatments do not always offer a better quality of life.

Clinic

Livingston Foundation Medical Center
3232 Duke Street
San Diego, CA 92110
Phone: 619-224-3515

Book

Hulda Regehr Clark, P.L.D., N.P., *The Cure for All Cancers: With 100 Case Histories* (San Diego, CA: New Century Press, 1993). This book is not about the Livingston program, but, like Livingston, the author claims that cancer is caused by a pathogen. An herbal remedy is offered.

Poultices

Historically, many people, including Native Americans and other indigenous peoples, have used poultices to draw tumors through the skin. I have heard of anecdotal success stories.

Book

Ingrid Naiman, *Cancer Salve and Suppositories: A Botanical Approach to Treatment* (Santa Fe, NM: Seventh Ray Press, 1997). This is a well-researched guide to this type of herbal medicine. It is available from the author at P.O. Box 31007, Santa Fe, NM 87594-1007. Phone: 505-473-5797.

Organization

Roots and Blossom Apothecary
Phone: 505-982-6360
Provides a catalog of herbs.

Shark and Bovine Cartilage

Shark cartilage has shown some effectiveness in slowing the growth of new blood vessels needed for tumor growth. A Cuban study that got good results used an intestinal infusion to introduce massive doses of shark cartilage into the patients. There is much less absorption when taken in pill form. I. William Lane, Ph.D., the chief proponent and one of the major manufacturers of shark cartilage, mentions in his book that a daily therapeutic dose of shark cartilage is one-third of a person's body weight in grams—i.e., a one hundred and fifty pound person would need 150/3 = 50 grams of shark cartilage. As with numerous supplements, many people do not know the therapeutic dose and may not be taking the correct amount. Practitioners using this treatment state that it must be used for two to four months to determine if it is working, and then it may need to be continued indefinitely. There is also some concern that the cartilage's effectiveness may be neutralized by stomach acids during digestion.

Of course, everyone claims their shark cartilage is of better quality than everyone else's, and Lane claims he has the only FDA-approved supplement.

Bovine cartilage, also known as Catrix, has been used medically for over twenty years, originally as a treatment for healing wounds. John Prudden, M.D., is a respected mainstream clinician who is often called the father of cartilage therapy. He refers to shark cartilage as his "illegitimate child" because his work spurred shark cartilage promoter Lane's interest and because he does not think shark cartilage is as effective as bovine cartilage. Dr. Prudden states that the ability of shark and bovine cartilage to inhibit the growth of new blood vessels for tumors is basically equivalent, but he does not think these survive the digestive process to a useful degree. He believes bovine cartilage works instead through stimulating the immune system. Bovine cartilage is four to ten times less expensive than shark cartilage and requires about one-eighth the therapeutic dosage. The December 1985 *Journal of Biological Response Modifiers* published Prudden's clinical results with thirty-one cancer patients who had failed to respond to standard therapies or had untreatable cancers. Patients normally started treatment with subcutaneous injections and then took 9 grams of cartilage daily, orally in 3-gram installments. Ninety percent of the patients had a partial or complete response. Eleven patients (35 percent) showed complete responses, eight patients (26 percent) had a complete response but sustained a relapse, six (19 percent) sustained a partial response, three (10 percent) a minimal response, and one patient showed no response.

Because cancer may or may not return after successful treatment, patients must continue taking the therapeutic dose of 9 grams daily to avoid a possible remission. Dr. Prudden states it can take up to four months for positive effects to appear if the therapy works. He also states he has never observed any toxicity from using bovine cartilage in the twenty-five years he has worked with it, even with doses that are three times the therapeutic dose.

Dr. Prudden has continued his research since his 1985 study. He will soon release the results of his work with over two hundred patients, which, he says, verify and exceed the results he published in 1985. He states bovine cartilage has shown effectiveness with some hard-to-cure cancers, including two brain cancers, non-small-cell cancer of the lung, and pancreatic cancer.

Book

William Lane, Ph.D., and Linda Comac, *Sharks Don't Get Cancer* (Garden City Park, NY: Avery Publishing Group, 1992), and *Sharks Still Don't Get Cancer* (Garden City Park, NY: Avery Publishing Group, 1996).

Article

John Prudden, M.D., "The Treatment of Human Cancer with Agents Prepared from Bovine Cartilage," *Journal of Biological Response Modifiers* 4 (Dec. 1985): 551–84.

Working Paper

Does Cartilage Cure Cancer? The Shark and Bovine Cartilage Controversy: An Independent Assessment. Working paper by Vivekan Don Flint and Michael Lerner. Available from Michael Lerner's Commonweal program and at their website: www.commonwealhealth.org.

Organizations

Phoenix Biologics
2794 Loker Avenue West, Suite 104
Carlsbad, CA 92008
Phone: 760-603-0542

Commonweal
P.O. Box 316

Bolinas, CA 94924
Phone: 415-868-0970

Practitioner

Dr. John Prudden
104 Post Office Road
Waccabuc, NY 10597
Phone: 914-763-5290

Compassionate Use: Acquiring Unapproved Therapies

The Compassionate Use Law or eIND (Emergency Investigational New Drug process) was supposed to make untested or unapproved therapies more readily available for terminal patients who had exhausted other treatments. My understanding is that the process varies from quick to lengthy and requires your physician to provide detailed information to the FDA. Even then your request may or may not be approved. Instead, most patients use the "personal importation policy" to acquire alternatives. If the substance is to be hand carried into the country, it must be for personal use, which means it can be no more than a reasonable three-month supply, and you must have a prescription, which may be from another country.

If you want to obtain substances by mail, again it must be no more than a three-month supply and be something that is unavailable in the United States. You must have a signed letter from a doctor on the doctor's letterhead stating the diagnosis of a life-threatening disease; that he or she recommends you take the drug because other common drugs were tried but failed, or that you were unable to take them for whatever reason; and that he or she will monitor your use of the substance. A copy of the letter is sent to the provider of the substance, who must include it with the product for review by a customs official who considers these shipments individually. Note that this procedure is allowed *only* for substances for which the FDA has not issued an import alert. Customs officials allow these substances through at their discretion. They will follow the FDA's suggestion in most cases. For substances with import alerts, the only sure way to receive treatment is to go in person.

Website

Food and Drug Administration: www.fda.gov

This website includes a complete list of FDA import alerts for all types of materials, in addition to health-related substances. Choose "Foods," then "Program Areas: Imports, Exports," then "Import alerts."

There is no separate category for cancer at the FDA website, and the site's search engine does not (as many do not) perform reliably. (For example, my search for 714-X found no matches, although 714-X has an import alert.) Since developing the website, the FDA no longer maintains a designated telephone number for obtaining a hard-copy list of substances with import alerts. I was told by the Division of Import Operations, the division of the FDA responsible for import alerts, that people without Web access could call them at 301-443-6553; or contact the consumer affairs offices at regional FDA offices listed in the FDA United States government listings in your phone book; or file a Freedom of Information request, by calling 301-443-6310 for information. I tried the first two suggestions without success.

It seems odd that we need to use the Freedom of Information Act to obtain the list of substances that the FDA doesn't want people to import.

Book

Beverly Zakarian, *The Activist Cancer Patient: How to Take Charge of Your Treatment* (New York: John Wiley & Sons, 1996). Has detailed information on obtaining treatments through the eIND process.

Organization

Office of Special Health Issues
Food and Drug Administration
5600 Fishers Lane (HF-12)
Rockville, MD 20857
Phone: 301-827-4460

Call or write this FDA office for information on, or for requesting treatments through, the eIND process.

Interview with Berkley Bedell, former U.S. Congressman

on His Experiences With Alternative Treatments for Cancer and on Setting Up the Office of Alternative Medicine

Berkley Bedell is on the advisory board of the Office of Alternative Medicine. He was a successful Iowa businessman who served six terms in Congress and retired in 1988 after contracting Lyme disease from a tick bite received while fishing. Convinced that his illness was healed by alternative medical treatments, he became actively involved in the investigation of alternative interventions, and after contracting prostate cancer, he treated himself with 714-X and believes it was responsible for his cure.

Bedell was the driving force behind the creation of the Office of Alternative Medicine at the National Institutes of Health and serves on its advisory board. He is the founder and president of the National Foundation of Alternative Medicine, an organization that investigates alternative treatments for disease worldwide.

Start by telling us what happened to you.

When I was in Congress, I contracted Lyme disease, and I was treated with conventional treatments three times. Each time, they would inject a strong antibiotic into my veins each day for twenty-one days or longer—one time, almost six weeks. And each time, I would feel better for a while, but then I'd get right back to where I was before. So, I finally turned to an alternative treatment.

That alternative treatment was colostrum, which is the first milk that comes when a mammal has offspring. After taking that for about three months, I no longer suffered from Lyme disease. The sad thing is that I get calls almost every day from people who have read about my recovery and want to know what I did. But that treatment is not available to them because under current FDA rules and regulations, you cannot market a drug unless you've gone through the FDA approval process. And they consider colostrum—which is milk—a *drug* if you're using it to cure a disease.

Then, at that time, I also came down with prostate cancer, and again I went through the conventional types of treatment. I had my prostate removed, but they "didn't get it all" and I had radiation. About two years after that, as a result of what I'd found with my Lyme disease, I made quite an effort to see what I could learn about alternative treatments. It appeared to me that many of these treatments really had some efficacy, but they were frozen out of our system because of the way our system operates.

So I went up to Quebec, Canada, to see this gentleman named Gaston Naessens. Mr. Naessens has built a microscope that he claims is more powerful than conventional light microscopes. With it, he claims he can see a series in a person's blood where the organisms he sees—which are not recognized by conventional medicine—go through a series of some thirteen growth cycles, from nonpathogenic organisms to pathogenic organisms. While I was there, I said, "Why don't you look at my blood and see if it looks all right?" He looked at it and he said, "Oh, I'm sorry, it doesn't."

He also claims that the cancer organism has a tremendous affinity for nitrogen and that one of the reasons that cancer grows and develops is that the cancer steals all the nitrogen so that your immune system does not have the nitrogen it needs to operate effectively. His treatment is an injection into your lymph area of a nitrogen-type compound that floods the area. I did that myself for twenty-one days and went back to him to look at my blood again. He said, "Your blood's clear now, but I think you ought to do it another twenty-one days." I did. That was four years ago, and at least all my blood tests and everything else indicate that I'm clear of my cancer.

I cannot guarantee that he was right in his diagnosis. All I can tell you is I've got friends who were in the same situation that I was in at that time, who are no longer with us today, and I'm alive and healthy, and I give credit to that treatment.

The result of all this has been that I have become primarily involved [in promoting] the investigation of alternative treatments for disease, particularly cancer, but also Alzheimer's and arthritis—diseases for which, I believe, conventional treatments are of limited effectiveness. Many of these [alternative practitioners] claim significant effectiveness for the treatments they're giving; I think it's criminal that we don't at least [try to] find out whether or not they are.

Most of [these practitioners] have a sound scientific logic as to why [their treatments] work. I believe we've got a completely closed system, where it costs millions and millions of dollars to go through the FDA approval process, which pretty well cuts out anybody except the large pharmaceutical companies in marketing any type of drug. So no one's going to spend millions of dollars to market something unless they can get a patent on it and charge a real high price for it.

It's my further belief that—I'm not a doctor—that pharmaceutical drugs and antibiotics are tremendously effective for all our infectious communicable diseases like chicken pox, mumps, measles, all that sort of thing. But we're finding they're not *nearly* as effective for our degenerative diseases, such as cancer, Alzheimer's, MS [multiple sclerosis], those sorts of things. It's terrible that we still say the *only* thing that's going to be able to get into the [medical] system is pharmaceutical drugs.

What did your conventional doctor think of all that?

I don't know what you mean by a conventional doctor, and I think that's where we get into trouble. Who is a conventional doctor, and who is an alternative practitioner? There are a great many doctors who would be considered conventional but who are using some of these alternative treatments. Frankly, they do so at the risk of getting in terrible, terrible difficulty; but I don't think that you can separate them quite that clearly. Certainly, the people I go to practice and are open to some of these alternative types of treatment, but I'm sure they're the minority. I don't think it's right to say, well, this is an alternative practitioner, and this is a conventional practitioner. I think there's a large and growing group sort of in the middle.

Do you have any suggestions on how to go about choosing an alternative treatment or treatments?

No, I don't have an opinion on how one should go about choosing what you should do. That's one of the problems I face: people call me all the time and ask, "What should I do?" And I am not in the position to advise them. Partly because I would not know *how* to advise them. And that's what I think is so wrong about our system: it would not be a big job to check out these alternative treatments objectively—not negatively, but objectively—to see how well they work and get the information out.

That's why I'm so excited about this Office of Alternative Medicine at the NIH, if we can ever get it really up and running. The protocol that we plan to use is simple: check the patients prior to their treatment to confirm the diagnosis, have the practitioner treat them, and check them after treatment to find out whether the treatment was effective or not. That's a very simple thing to do. It's an inexpensive thing to do. And my argument is that it's the first thing you should do.

Under current practices at the National Cancer Institute, if someone has a treatment that they think is effective, and if they can convince the National Cancer Institute to look at it—and as far as I know, they've only run full tests on three alternative treatments since they've been in operation—[the NCI] takes that treatment to somebody else, like Sloan-Kettering [Memorial Sloan-Kettering Institute for Cancer Research, New York] or Mayo Clinic [in Rochester, Minnesota], and asks, "Will you see if it works?" But my argument is that Sloan or Mayo might do things differently than the original practitioner did who made it work. If they come back with a report that it didn't work, that's pretty well the end of that treatment.

The first thing I think we ought to find out is whether there is a practitioner who can effectively treat brain cancer, or whatever else it may be, and then [we ought to] go to somebody else to have them try it, allowing the practitioner who claims success to supervise how it's done. It appears to me that what we've got is a system that's almost opposed to trying to find out what works and what doesn't work, compared to a system that would say, Let's see if there's anything out there that can help us develop more effective treatment and a better understanding of disease.

Why is this problem of researching alternative treatments difficult for the National Cancer Institute, while the Office of Alternative Medicine seems to find a way to do it so easily?

I think it's a mind-set. You have a group of scientists who think they know more than anybody else and who do not want anybody challenging their thinking and their beliefs. I come from a business background, and the main reason our business was successful was because of our research efforts. It was a fishing tackle business, and we built better fishing equipment than other people. But two of our three major items are not ones that we discovered and developed; they were ideas that had come from outside and that we improved upon. My big argument with the National Cancer Institute is that it's cloistered. It sits there by itself doing a bunch of research without getting out and looking at what other people are doing to see if they can learn from it. The sad thing about that is that other countries are substantially ahead of us in many of these areas, while the great creativity generally is in the United States. This creativity in America is what's brought us forward so much. But in medicine, in my opinion, it's absolutely squelched.

Tell us a little more about the Office of Alternative Medicine—what it is, how you got involved, and why you think it's important.

I happen to be a friend of Senator Tom Harkin, whom I talked to about what I had found and my beliefs and so on. And Senator Harkin, chairman of the Health Appropriations subcommittee of the Senate, put two million dollars into the NIH budget for the establishment of an Office of Alternative Medicine. Harkin's legislation called for an advisory committee, which I now serve on, to be established to advise that office. It has been a very difficult, slow job with the bureaucracy, getting the committee really going the way I would like to see it go. But it looks like we're finally getting there.

The purpose of the office, as it was stated in the report on Harkin's legislation, was to "investigate and validate these treatments." That's what I think is not being done generally by NIH. It might be that some of those treatments are not perfect but that they're better than what we have. Or there might be two of them that use somewhat similar science. And we would say, "Well, how does this fit in, and what can we learn from this?" Or it might be that we would find out that Mr. Naessens's theory of these tiny, tiny organisms that have particular properties is true, and it might help us change completely how we look at cancer and other diseases. Second,

I believe we should open up the system more. As long as the treatment is nontoxic, as long as there are no false claims made about the treatment, as long as the patient is completely advised as to what the treatment is, and as long as the patient signs a statement saying they want to be treated with that intervention, it seems to me [that we should let people] be treated with it. [Let them try] colostrum, which is really milk, if they wish to do so, to see if it would work. [It's a shame] when they send people home; conventional medicine says, "I'm sorry, there's nothing we can do for you, you can go home and die." It seems an awful shame if the patient knows somebody who has been to Europe and was successfully treated, but the patient doesn't have the money to go to Europe, so he or she has to say, "Well, I guess I've got to home and die." Even if it's a 10 percent chance, it's sure a lot better to have a 10 percent chance than a 0 percent chance.

In what kind of situation would you recommend that somebody look into an alternative treatment for cancer, as opposed to just going to a standard medical doctor?

First of all, everyone has to understand I'm not a doctor. It's really not proper for me to tell people what they should do if they have a malignancy. I *can* tell you that I'm awfully glad that *I* did, that I looked at these treatments for both my Lyme disease and my malignancy, rather than saying, "Well, surely the doctor must know best."

Is there one message that you would give to somebody with cancer?

I guess my message as a layman, particularly to someone who had terminal cancer and whose doctor sent them home saying, "You only have this long to live, and there's nothing more we can do for you," is not to take that advice. I would urge them to look at the different alternative treatments that might be available. Because I can tell you that there are people who have turned to some of these alternative treatments and are now alive, well, and healthy. I don't think it's a guarantee, but I sure would not accept that diagnosis if it were given to me.

[All interviews have been edited for length and clarity.]

Berkeley Bedell is the founder and President of the National Foundation for Alternative Medicine. The Foundation can be contacted at:

1155 Connecticut Ave., N. W., Suite 300
Washington, D.C. 20036
Phone: 202-429-6633

5

Complementary and Supplemental Therapies

Complementary treatments are used to supplement your primary treatment, not to replace it. These therapies range from mind-body interventions such as psychotherapy, meditation, and imagery, to bodywork such as massage and acupressure, to foods and supplements that you ingest to aid physical body processes, such as vitamins and minerals. Some alternative treatments, such as the original Gerson diet (see "Gerson Therapy," chapter 4), can also be used as complementary treatments. In this chapter we will cover the most common foods, diets, vitamins, supplements, and bodywork techniques that people with cancer have found helpful. Mind-body interventions are addressed in Part 3.

Acupuncture

Acupuncture is an ancient Chinese healing art based on the idea that the body's proper functioning depends on the unrestricted flow of life force or energy, called *chi* or *qi* (pronounced "chee"). Disease is said to develop from imbalances, blocks, or restrictions in the flow of this vital energy. Acupuncture needles are placed at points in energy pathways called *meridians* to stimulate and restore movement of the energy.

Richard P. Magdaleno, O.M.D., a Connecticut-based acupuncturist, describes this therapy:

Recently, science has determined that human beings are complex bioelectric systems. This understanding has been the foundation of acupuncture practice for several thousands of years. Energy circulates throughout the body along well-defined pathways. Points on the skin along these pathways are energetically connected to specific organs, body structures, and systems. If this energy circulation is disrupted, optimum function is affected, and this results in pain or illness. Acupuncture points are stimulated to balance the circulation of energy, which influences the health of the entire being.

For treating cancer, Chinese medicine uses both acupuncture and herbs (see "Chinese and Western Herbal Medicine," in this chapter). My impression of acupuncture as well as of some other subtle energy techniques is that if you choose this path, start early; later in the game, I think you need a bigger hammer.

This viewpoint is corroborated by Richard Walters in his book *Options: The Alternative Cancer Therapy Book* (see below):

"In China, surgery, chemotherapy, and radiation are considered viable treatments for benign and malignant tumors by physicians who are attempting to integrate Eastern and Western methods. Conventional treatments may be required to deal with a situation within the time available to the patient," notes Zhang Dai-Zhao, a specialist in cancer treatment in Beijing. Although Chinese energetic therapies such as herbal medicine and acupuncture may be able to eventually dismantle pathologic matter, "they may take more time than the patient has," he states. Many practitioners in China say that the best results against cancer are obtained by means of a joint attack combining Oriental and Western medicine, with the patient pursuing a suitable diet, Chinese yoga, and therapeutic exercise.

Books

Richard Walters, *Options: The Alternative Cancer Therapy Book* (Garden City Park, NY: Avery Publishing Group, 1993).

Michael Lerner, Ph.D., *Choices in Healing: Integrating the Best of Conventional and Complementary Approaches to Cancer* (Cambridge, MA: MIT Press, 1994). Can be viewed at the Commonweal website: www.commonwealhealth.org.

Organization

American Association of Oriental Medicine
433 Front Street
Catasauqua, PA 18032
Phone: 610-433-2448
Provides referrals to acupuncturists near you.

Bodywork:
Massage, Reflexology, and Acupressure

The body's natural response to stress and emotions is to tighten physically. This not only makes you uncomfortable, it also impedes the natural flow of energy and the proper functioning of internal organs. Therapeutic massage is a wonderful gift to yourself to help relieve stress and feel better.

Reflexology is a massage of the foot's pressure points. Pressure points are spots that, according to the discipline, correspond to all the different organs and parts of our body. By applying pressure and massaging these points, healing chi energy is stimulated and circulated, as it is in acupuncture and acupressure. If you cannot afford massage or professional reflexology, you can roll your foot on a foot roller or a hand ball and imagine your breath moving oxygen into the sore spots you find on the bottom of your feet.

Acupressure is similar to acupuncture but without needles. Specific pressure points are massaged with the tips of the fingers to create a small electrical charge, which establishes and equalizes the flow of energy through the meridians, or energy pathways. You can learn the basics of acupressure and apply them yourself.

Although these techniques obviously will not cure your cancer, they can certainly help relieve the stress cancer causes, and, if the Chinese are correct, they may promote the body's overall health.

Chi-kung or Qigong

Chi-kung is a system of body movement, breathing, and visualization that was a healing art preceding the evolution of its martial art derivative, tai chi. Through specific movements, the vital energy of the body, or "chi force," is cleansed, cultivated, balanced, and then circulated and applied to assist healing.

Books

David Eisenberg, M.D., et al., "Unconventional Medicine in the United States," *New England Journal of Medicine* 328 (Jan. 28, 1993): 246–51. Provides one Western doctor's experience of Eastern medicine.

W. John Diamond, M.D., and W. Lee Cowden, M.D., with Burton Goldberg, *An Alternative Medicine Definitive Guide to Cancer* (Tiburon, CA: Future Medicine Publishing, 1997). This contains a brief introduction to qigong exercises.

Organization

International Society for the Study of Subtle Energy Medicine
356 Goldco Circle
Golden, CO 80403
Phone: 303-425-4625

Chinese and Western Herbal Medicine

One of the oldest medical treatments is the therapeutic use of plants, known as herbal medicine. It is the primary element of many forms of folk, traditional, Native American, and Chinese medicines. More than three thousand different plant species have been used to treat cancer worldwide and also have been the source of several conventional chemotherapeutic drugs. Herbal medicine, not acupuncture, is the primary intervention of Chinese medicine, contrary to what most Westerners think.

The following description is from *Alternative Medicine: Expanding Medical Horizons,* a report that was sponsored by the Office of Alternative Medicine (Washington, DC: GPO, 1994, stock no. 017-040-00537-7), which contains an excellent overview of alternative and complementary approaches, including Chinese medicine.

[In Chinese herbal medicine] medications are classified according to their energetic qualities (e.g., heating, cooling, moisturizing, drying) and prescribed for their action on corresponding organ dysfunction, energy disorders, disturbed internal energy, blockage of the meridians, or seasonal physical demands. One unique aspect of traditional prescribing is the use of complex mixtures containing many ingredients. Such prescriptions are systematically compounded to have several effects: to principally affect the disease or disharmony, to balance out any potential side effects of the principal therapy, and to direct the therapy to a specific area or a physical process in the body.

Michael Lerner, founder of the Commonweal program, is well known for research-based evaluations of cancer therapies. According to Lerner, in his book *Choices in Healing: Integrating the Best of Conventional and Complementary Approaches to Cancer* (Cambridge, MA: MIT Press, 1994), "If anything, most practitioners (there certainly are exceptions) of traditional Chinese medicine can—on the basis of the research literature—be criticized for understating the promise of their treatments for cancer." To explore this avenue of treatment, one clearly needs to find a qualified Chinese medicine practitioner, which may be easier in some geographic areas than others. Lerner goes on to state:

Traditional Chinese medicine is, in my judgment, one of the most intriguing of the adjunctive therapies for cancer. There is considerable evidence for its benefits in pain control and in alleviating the side effects of chemotherapy and radiation therapy. Patients frequently report these benefits, as well. There are also some reasons to believe that traditional Chinese medicine may help in the battle to extend life with cancer and to lower the risk of recurrence of cancer.

Recently, herbology has taken root in the health food and self-care movements, with much publicity about the immune-enhancing properties of many herbs like astragalus, echinacea, cat's claw, and green tea. Astragalus and green tea have been the subject of the most cancer-related research. Astragalus is a nontoxic herb whose derivatives have been shown to boost immunity, fight cancer, and protect against some side effects of chemotherapy. Green tea has been the subject of much research in Japan, where researchers have isolated the chemical gallocatechin gallate (EGCG), which was shown to inhibit tumors in the skin, lungs, and in the intestines of mice. More recently, a study in the December 17, 1997, *Journal of the National Cancer Institute* demonstrated EGCG's effectiveness at killing human cancer cells in laboratory experiments.

Research like this, preliminary as it is, plus the belief that Japan's low lung cancer rate may be due to the consumption of copious amounts of green tea, has made this unfermented tea a popular beverage with smokers.

Consultation with a professional herbalist can help you determine how herbs are best used. For example, after herbs are used for a period of time, a "rest" period is often recommended when herbs are not taken. Although there have been few reported side effects with use of most of these popular herbs, it is best to consult with a qualified professional herbalist, and your doctor, about any known problems with combining herbs and medications.

Books

Michael Lerner, Ph.D., *Choices in Healing: Integrating the Best of Conventional and Complementary Approaches to Cancer* (Cambridge, MA: MIT Press, 1994). Can be viewed at the Commonweal website: www.commonwealhealth.org.

Hong-Yen Hsu, *Treating Cancer with Chinese Herbs* (New Canaan, CT: Keats Publishing, 1993).

Ralph W. Moss, Ph.D., *Cancer Therapy: The Independent Consumer's Guide to Nontoxic Treatment and Prevention* (New York: Equinox Press, 1992).

Dai-zhao Zhang, *Treatment of Cancer by Integrated Chinese-Western Medicine* (Boulder, CO: Blue Poppy Press, 1989).

Report

Office of Alternative Medicine, *Alternative Medicine: Expanding Medical Horizons* (Washington, DC: Government Printing Office, 1994). Stock no. 017-040-00537-7.

Working Paper

Herbal Remedies for Cancer, by Vivekan Don Flint and Michael Lerner.

Available from Michael Lerner's Commonweal program and at their website: www.commonwealhealth.org.

Organization

Commonweal
P.O. Box 316
Bolinas, CA 94924
Phone: 415-868-0970
Website: www.commonwealhealth.org

Information

The World Research Foundation cancer research package includes much information on Chinese medicine as well as large amounts of information on other approaches, for a reasonable fee (see "Research Services," under "Chapter Resources" at the end of this chapter).

Chlorella

Chlorella is a green algae rich in proteins, vitamins, nucleic acids, and the highest content of chlorophyll of any plant. In humans, chlorophyll is a potent blood builder and detoxifier.

Like PSK (see "Polysaccharide Krestin," below), chlorella also contains polysaccharides, which induce antitumor activity in a variety of cancers in experiments with mice. It is available in health food stores.

Source

Health and Happiness Publishing
Fax: 800-694-2224

Offers *The Chlorella Source Book*, a binder full of research articles, available for a small fee.

Cleansing Techniques and Detoxification

Treatments that successfully break down a tumor mass, like chemotherapy and radiation, release dead cancer cells into the bloodstream.

It is well known that this necrotic material can overburden the body's cleansing organs and that these accumulated toxins pose a serious health threat to cancer patients.

Coffee enemas, like those used in the Gerson and Kelly/Gonzalez programs, are meant to deal with this problem (see "Gerson Therapy" and "Kelly/Gonzalez Program" in chapter 4). Coffee enemas consist of a solution of one quart of water and two tablespoons of normally brewed, preferably organic, coffee. Enemas keep material moving through the intestines and help cleanse toxins from the bowel. Coffee stimulates the release of toxins from the liver and gallbladder. The liver is the body organ essential for removing toxins from the blood.

Fortunately, there are less intrusive and easier cleansing methods that may work as well. Many natural high-quality herbal cleansing and bowel rejuvenation supplements are available from health food stores and are recommended for detoxification and whenever bowel movements are impeded. Some advocates of detoxification techniques maintain that enemas are necessary to keep up with the large release of toxins and cancer cells that are being killed off while undergoing cancer treatment.

Antibiotics given to cancer patients to help them avoid infections also kill friendly bacteria needed for proper bowel function. Replenishing the bowel with acidophilus and other "good" bacteria can be helpful. Health food stores also carry formulas and herbs like Hepato-Pure and milk thistle to detoxify and help maintain liver and kidney function.

Liver-cleansing foods include beets, carrots, lemons, parsnips, dandelion greens, watercress, and burdock root.

Books

Linda Berry, *Internal Cleansing: Rid Your Body of Toxins and Return to Vibrant Health* (Rocklin, CA: Prima Publishing, 1997).

James F. Balch, M.D., and Phyllis A. Balch, C.N.C., *Prescription for Nutritional Healing: A Practical A–Z Reference* (Garden City Park, NY: Avery Publishing Group, 1997). Although not cancer specific, this book includes information on detoxification regimens.

Diet

Diet alone is only occasionally claimed to bring about a cancer cure, but there is little doubt that diet and nutrition can play a large role in aiding the restoration of the body's immune system and in dealing with the effects of cancer and its treatment. The resources here provide general introductions to and personal stories about using diet to help heal from cancer.

Books

Eydie Mae Hunsberger, with Chris Loeffter, *How I Conquered Cancer Naturally* (Garden City Park, NY: Avery Publishing Group, 1992).

Ruth Jochems and Linus Pauling, *Dr. Moerman's Anti-Cancer Diet: Holland's Revolutionary Nutritional Program for Combating Cancer* (Garden City Park, NY: Avery Publishing Group, 1990).

Maureen B. Keane and Daniella Chace, *What to Eat If You Have Cancer: A Guide to Adding Nutritional Therapy to Your Treatment Plan* (Chicago, IL: Contemporary Books, 1996).

Annemarie Colbin, *Food & Healing,* rev. ed. (New York: Ballantine Books, 1996).

Usha Lad and Vasant Lad, *Ayurvedic Cooking for Self-Healing*, 2d ed. (Albuquerque, NM: Ayurvedic Press, 1997).

Diet: Macrobiotics

Yukikazu Sakurazawa, who was better known in the West as George Ohsawa, described the principles of Oriental medicine and philosophy under the name of "macrobiotics." His teachings inspired Michio Kushi, whose name has since become synonymous with macrobiotics and its teaching. Kushi is the founder of the East-West Foundation, a nonprofit organization dedicated to educating people about the benefits of macrobiotics. The macrobiotic lifestyle is based on whole and natural foods, and it has resulted in cures for some cancer patients. The central elements in the diet are cooked vegetables and whole grains; there are other numerous dietary restrictions and recommendations.

Organization

Kushi Institute
P.O. Box 7
Becket, MA 01223-0007
Phone: 413-623-5741

Books

Michio Kushi with Edward Esko, *The Macrobiotic Approach to Cancer: Towards Preventing Cancer with Diet and Lifestyle* (Garden City Park, NY: Avery Publishing Group, 1991).

Michio Kushi with Edward Esko, *The Macrobiotic Cancer-Prevention Cookbook* (Wayne, NJ: Avery Publishing Group, 1988).

Diet: Metabolic Programs

The word *metabolic* pertains to metabolism, the complex process by which the body breaks down foodstuffs and vitamins into necessary physical components. Not specifically cancer treatments in themselves, metabolic programs aim at restoring the body to its proper metabolism, nutritional balance, and overall functioning.

Metabolic practitioners maintain that people use nutrition differently depending on their specific type of metabolism. They first ascertain the individual's metabolic type, then use an individualized program of vitamins, supplements, natural health foods, diet, and detoxification to balance body chemistry. The rationale is that, when body imbalances are repaired, the body is better able to deal with any disease, since disease is usually the result of an imbalance. One long-time proponent of metabolic "host repair" programs is Ruth Sackman, founder and director of the nonprofit resource organization Foundation for the Advancement of Cancer Therapy. She says, "Our position is that the body chemistry is out of order, that the body itself is not controlling the problem, it's producing the abnormal cells, and it is not stopping the production just because there's a surgical procedure that removes the tumor itself and discards it. You have to correct the broken-down body function."

Metabolic practitioners were among the first people in the alternative health field to recognize that people metabolize vitamins differently. Instead of the shotgun approach of taking all vitamins and hoping for the best, metabolic practitioners began to tailor vitamins and supplements to the individual body chemistries of their patients. As the understanding of different metabolic types increases, so does the complexity of the topic. In this field, using a trained consultant is recommended.

Organization

Foundation for Advancement in Cancer Therapy
P.O. Box 1242
Old Chelsea Station
New York, NY 10113
Phone: 212-741-2790

Provides information and referrals, emphasizes metabolic, biologic, and nutritional approaches that can be used either as supplemental or as an alternative to orthodox treatment.

Practitioners

Jack Taylor, M.S., D.C.
3606 Algonquin Road, Suite 801
Rolling Meadows, IL 60008
Phone: 847-222-1192

Healthexcell
277 West Chewuch Road
Winthrop, WA 98862
Phone: 509-996-2131
Website: www.healthexcel.com

Provider of a metabolic program. Cost for initial evaluation is approximately $300.

Diet: Organic Foods

Organic foods are foods that are all natural, have not been irradiated, and have no chemical additives. For people trying to heal cancer, chemical additives are thought to be just one more foreign substance that can stress your body's systems. The reasoning is that eliminating things that stress the body enables the immune system to spend more of its energy fighting cancer.

Enzymes

Enzymes are catalysts for either building up or breaking down molecules. They are used to digest food, especially proteins. The breaking down of proteins results in amino acids, which become neurotransmitters, hormones, and antibodies, which fulfill a variety of roles in the glands and organs of the body.

It is believed that some enzymes help remove the fibrin coating of cells, exposing antigens on the cancer cell surface that identify it as a target for the immune system. This also reduces the adhesiveness, or stickiness, of cells and may reduce the ability of cancer cells to adhere to other areas of the body or to metastasize.

Taking oral supplements of enzymes, except for those like pepsin, used by the stomach, was once thought useless. Enzymes were believed not to survive the journey through the stomach to the small intestines, where they are used to break down proteins into amino acids. Research has indicated that this is not so, according to R. Michael Williams, M.D., Ph.D., a traditionally trained oncologist and immunologist.

Dr. Williams, senior medical director and chief medical officer and cofounder of Cancer Treatment Centers of America and coauthor of *Enzymes: The Fountain of Life* (Charleston, SC: Neville Press, 1994), recommends that his cancer patients take a multiple enzyme supplement. One such supplement is Wobenzym or Wobenzym N (they are the same formula), available through most health food stores as well as through the distributor Marlyn Nutraceuticals.

Dr. Williams takes fifteen of these multiple enzyme supplements daily as part of his own wellness program and recommends his cancer patients take up to thirty daily, one to two hours before meals, with eight ounces of water. Digestive enzyme supplements, which often contain some of the same enzymes as the Wobenzym combination, are meant to be taken with meals to aid in the predigestion of food in the stomach.

Books

W. John Diamond, M.D., W. Lee Cowden, M.D., with Burton Golberg, *An Alternative Medicine Definitive Guide to Cancer* (Tiburon, CA: Future Medicine Publishing, 1997). Contains a useful summary of enzyme information.

D. A. Lopez, M.D., R. Michael Williams, M.D., Ph.D, and K. Miehlke, M.D., *Enzymes: The Fountain of Life* (Charleston, SC: Neville Press, 1994). This book can be ordered from Natural Resources at www.true-health.com or from:

Infinity 2
Infinity Towers
63 E. Main Street, #700
Mesa, AZ 85201

Supplier

Marlyn Nutraceuticals
14851 N. Scottsdale Road
Scottsdale, AZ 85254
Phone: 800-222-4405

Enzymatic Therapy
825 Challenger Drive
Green Bay, WI 59311
Phone: 800-783-2286

Offers a high-potency proteolytic enzyme similar to Wobenzym under the name of Mega-Zyme.

Essential Fatty Acids

Omega-3 (alpha-linolenic acid) and omega-6 (linoleic acid) are essential fatty acids. Essential nutrients are those needed but not made by the body, and therefore they must come from an outside food source. Studies indicate that higher levels of omega-6 may increase the risk of cancer, while higher levels of omega-3 can have anticancer effects. Omega-6 oils are readily available in an American diet, but omega-3 is seriously lacking. One reason for this is omega-3 is an unstable oil that spoils easily and is taken out of foods to increase their shelf life.

The German biochemist Johanna Budwig, Ph.D., who discovered essential fatty acids, developed an anticancer diet that consists of 40 grams of flaxseed oil, rich in omega-3, 100 grams of skim milk, and 25 grams of milk (1 oz. = 28 grams). Many patients experienced tumor reduction within three months, and some showed even more dramatic results. Flaxseed-oil supplementation deserves exploration as a complementary therapy. A few quality oil brands are Omega, Barlene's, and Udo's Choice.

Books

Johanna Budwig, Ph.D., *Flax Oil as a True Aid Against Arthritis, Heart Infarction, Cancer, and Other Diseases* (Vancouver, BC: Apple Publishing, 1996).

Johanna Budwig, Ph.D., *The Oil Protein Diet Cookbook: Use of Oils in Cooking* (Vancouver, BC: Apple Publishing, 1996).

Ross Pelton, Ph.D., and Lee Overholser, Ph.D., *Alternatives in Cancer Therapy: The Complete Guide to Nontraditional Treatments* (New York: Simon & Schuster, 1994).

Provider

Dr. Johanna Budwig
Hegelstrasse 3
72250 Freundenstadt
Germany
Phone: 011-49-744-1766-7
Fax: 011-49-744-1851-25

Essiac Tea

Essiac is an Ojibwa Indian recipe given to Canadian nurse Rene Cassie. It is a combination of the herbs burdock root, sheep sorrel, slippery elm, and rhubarb root. Consumed as a tea, essiac is reported to have caused some remissions in hard-to-treat cancers.

Later in life, Cassie worked with respected international Dr. Charles Brusch (personal physician to John F. Kennedy) and supposedly improved the formula. The original formula is being distributed as "Essiac" to health food stores by Respirin Corporation. The supposedly improved formula, developed by Brusch, is being sold as "Flor-essence." These Essiac formulations are sold in health food stores without any references to cancer, to comply with FDA regulations.

Suppliers

Great Cape Cod Herb, Spice and Tea Co.
P.O. Box 1206
Brewster, MA 02631
Phone: 508-896-5900

Offers a reasonably priced essiac formula.

Herbal Advantage
Route 3, Box 92
Rogersville, MO 65742
Phone: 800-753-9199

Good source for reasonably priced herbs.

Website

www.znet.com/~oct31/essiac/index.shtml

Ginseng

Ginseng is considered to be a miracle herb, and research has just scratched the surface of its many properties. Ginseng is considered to be an adaptogen, a substance that assists the body systems and functioning to return to their natural state of balance. One of ginseng's many qualities is its ability to provide additional energy by increasing the blood's ability to carry oxygen and the life force, or *prana,* as it is called in Hindu and yogic traditions. As with other vitamins and supplements, there is a big difference in quality. Fraud is commonplace, with some suppliers offering a very low quality product consisting mostly of filler.

The effects of ginseng, if it is good, can usually be felt in three to four days of taking it once or twice a day; but can take from one to eight weeks to build up in your system. It is recommended that you take it in the morning and midafternoon; otherwise you may have trouble sleeping. The nice thing about ginseng is that, unlike coffee, it does not make you tired when it wears off.

Quality is best assured in root form. Soften the root by heating it in a pan over low heat, then slice it. Let the slice dissolve in your mouth. Or put it up in between your cheek and gum to allow it to leech slowly into your system. Less-expensive ginseng root can be found in herbal shops in Chinese communities. If root is unavailable or is too costly locally, look for the compound with a Korean government seal. The Korean government regulates its ginseng, and it has consistent good quality. Ginseng, although not a cure, has health benefits and may certainly help you feel better.

Working Paper

Herbal Remedies for Cancer, by Vivekan Don Flint and Michael Lerner. Includes an excellent review of ginseng-related research. Available from Michael Lerner's Commonweal program and at their website: www.commonwealhealth.org.

Haelan 851

Haelan 851 is a concentrated soy beverage from China. Used in China primarily as an complementary cancer treatment, it has high concentrations of genisteins, believed to be one of the prominent healing elements within soybeans. The product is very expensive and tastes terrible, but if the extravagant healing claims are factual, it may be worth looking into. The Internet would be a good place to locate people who have tried this to learn about their experiences. A package of research reports on soybean concentrate and cancer is available from United States Research reports; phone 800-275-4530. A similar concentrated product called Mega-Soy is available from the Life Extension Foundation.

Suppliers

Haelan Products
18568 142nd Ave N.E., Bldg. F
Woodinville, WA 98072
Phone 800-542-3526

Life Extension Foundation
995 S.W. 24th Street
Fort Lauderdale, FL 33315
Phone: 800-841-5433

Hydrazine Sulfate

Hydrazine sulfate is an unproven therapy, embroiled in debate over its effectiveness. Yet it is worth mentioning because it has helped many cancer patients with cachexia. Cachexia is the weight loss and wasting-away syndrome that is estimated to kill 40 percent of cancer patients before the cancer does. Hydrazine sulfate is a common, inexpensive, industrial chemical. Its use was pioneered by Joseph Gold, M.D., of the Syracuse Cancer Research Institute. Some studies have shown it to have anticancer effects, while others have indicated no benefit. It is not an approved treatment, but some doctors and patients are using it on an experimental basis.

Practitioner

Joseph Gold, M.D.
Syracuse Cancer Center
600 East Genesee Street
Syracuse, NY 13202
Phone: 315-472-6616

Supplier

Great Lakes Metabolics
1724 Hiawatha Court, N.E.
Rochester, MN 55906
Phone: 507-288-2348

Inositol Hexaphosphate (IP-6)

Inositol is a common constituent of seeds, grains, soybeans, fruits, and vegetables. An active component that has been the subject of research into its anticancer effects is inositol hexaphosphate or IP-6, also known as phytic acid. According to Dr. A. Shamsuddin, professor of pathology at the University of Maryland School of Medicine and former senior scientist at the National Cancer Institute, more than two dozen animal and in vitro (test tube) studies on human cancers have demonstrated IP-6's anticancer effects. In one study cancerous mice had an approximately 100 percent increase in natural killer cell activity when given inositol and IP-6 together.

Articles

A. Shamsuddin, M.D., "Comparison of Pure Inositol Hexaphosphate and High Bran Diet in the Prevention of DMBA-Induced Rat Mammary Carcinogenesis," *Nutrition and Cancer* 28 (1997): 7–13.

A. Shamsuddin, M.D., et al., "Minireview IP-6: A Novel Anti-Cancer Agent," *Live Science* 61 (1987): 343–54.

Suppliers

IP-6 is available in health food stores as Cell Forte, an Enzymatic Therapy product, with no claims as to its anticancer effects.

Enzymatic Therapy
825 Challenger Drive
Green Bay, WI 59311
Phone: 800-783-2286

Oxygen

Half a century ago, a German biochemist, Otto Warburg, found that cancer cells grow favorably in low-oxygen conditions, and since then research has shown that cancer cells do not survive in high-oxygen environments. It would seem logical, then, to avoid factors that deplete oxygen in the body, like smoking, and pursue those that enhance it. This may be one reason why juiced wheat grass is potentially helpful, as it is supposed to wash the blood with oxygen and chlorophyll.

Researcher Maurice Finkel, in his book *Fresh Hope in Cancer: Natural Methods for Prevention, Treatment, and Control of Cancer* (N. Devon, England: Health Science Press, 1978), reports that saturated fats and their by-products combine with oxygen, reducing oxygen levels in the body. He also states that fluoride inhibits cell respiration through its inactivation of magnesium, and he recommends avoiding fluoridated water. B vitamins are thought to be necessary for proper oxygen aerobiosis, and supplements like ginseng and CoQ10 enhance oxygen levels.

Stephen Fulder, in his book *How to Survive Medical Treatment: A Holistic Guide to Avoiding the Risks and Side Effects of Conventional Medicine* (Woodstock, NY: Beekman Publishers, 1995), reports that Russian researchers found that when animals with a particular type of cancer underwent an abdominal operation, the percentage of animals whose cancer spread normally increased from forty-nine to seventy-eight percent. If they were given Siberian ginseng, a supplement known to increase the oxygen level in blood, "there was no increase in metastasis as a result of the operation."

Oxygen-based therapies like hydrogen peroxide and ozone therapies, while discredited by conventional medicine, are backed by some credible research and proponents who advocate their use as anticancer agents. "Stabilized oxygen" products like Dioxychor and Aerobic 07 are oxygen-enhancing supplements currently available through some health food stores and catalogs.

Books

Ed McCabe, *Oxygen Therapies: A New Way of Approaching Disease* (Morrisvillle, NY: Energy Publications, 1988). This is the classic original on oxygen therapy and is a good starting point. The book and a catalog of information and supplements is available from the following organization.

Nathaniel Altman, *Oxygen Healing Therapies for Optimum Health and Vitality* (Rochester, VT: Healing Arts Press, 1995).

Organization

International Bioxidation Medicine Foundation
P.O. Box 891954
Oklahoma City, OK 73189
Phone: 405-478-4266

Website

Cancer Prevention and Treatment—Oxygen: www.canceranswer.com

Polysaccharide Krestin (PSK)

Polysaccharide Krestin (PSK) is an extract of the mushroom *Coriolis versicolor*, also known as *tramates versicolor*. It is an approved anticancer drug in Japan, where supposedly 20 percent of the total national expenditure on cancer agents is spent on PSK.

In more than sixty clinical studies, PSK demonstrated significant survival benefits for various cancers when used in combination with radiation or chemotherapy.

Suppliers

JHS Natural Products
P.O. Box 50398
Eugene, OR 97405
Phone: 541-344-1396

Connecticut Center for Health
87 Bennie O'Rourke Drive
Middletown, CT 06457
Phone: 860-347-8600

Vitamins

Many positive results from using vitamins have been demonstrated through research, although debate about their effectiveness remains. Independent laboratory tests indicate that our food sources no longer contain the same levels of vitamins that the government measured in them decades ago. It appears that agribusiness, by growing the same crops in the same ground, has depleted the soil and reduced the vitamin content of everyday vegetables.

The "recommended daily amount" (RDA) established by the government is a minimum standard based on what is believed to be needed in order to prevent illness. It is not based on requirements for optimal body functioning. Unfortunately, there is limited research on optimal nutrient levels and on vitamin absorption.

Another problem is that many vitamins and minerals can have conflicting effects when taken together, and in some cases the total effect is less than positive. In one study, beta-carotene was thought to worsen lung cancer. Unfortunately, of the countless numbers of interactions possible, most are unknown. For example, zinc, another mineral important to cell growth and regulation, may inhibit the action of selenium in doses exceeding 20 milligrams per day.

Michael Lerner's book *Choices in Healing: Integrating the Best of Conventional and Complementary Approaches to Cancer* (Cambridge, MA: MIT Press, 1994) contains an excellent synopsis of pertinent vitamin considerations for cancer patients and some of the most important research on vitamins.

If you plan to use vitamins, you may wish to consult a holistically oriented nutritionist or, better yet, a naturopathic physician (N.D.). Some nutritionists are conservatively trained and have been exposed only to conventional nutritional information sources. Ideally, you want unbiased professionals who are open to all potential help. Naturopaths are trained in natural healing techniques and nutrition, and if you find a good one, she or he can provide state-of-the-art information on vitamin supplementation. Naturopaths are covered by insurance in some states.

Some studies suggest cancer may recur with less frequency in someone taking supplements. One study with positive results was reported in the January 1994 *Journal of Urology*. Patients with bladder cancer were given BCG, an immune therapy, and large doses of zinc and vitamins A, B_6, C, and E. In ten months, 80 percent of the control group had a recurrence of cancer, while only 40 percent of those receiving extra vitamins had a recurrence of tumors.

It is virtually impossible to make recommendations that are valid for all people, yet it does seem prudent to take some vitamins, as it would appear that the potential benefits outweigh any drawbacks. Ralph Moss, Ph.D., author of *Cancer Therapy: The Independent Consumer's Guide to Nontoxic Treatment and Prevention* (New York: Equinox Press, 1992), in his interview for the documentary *Cancer: Increasing Your Odds for Survival,* recommended basic vitamin supplementation:

> The key ones, in terms of cancer, are Vitamins A, C, and E. [Vitamin] A can be taken in the form of beta-carotene, which is totally nontoxic, whereas vitamin A itself, in very high doses, could be toxic, but that rarely happens. In addition, the mineral selenium is depleted in a lot of soils where food is grown. Consequently, we may not be getting enough selenium, and it's prudent to take a little bit extra of that. These vitamins are known to be scavengers of free radicals, which are harmful chemicals generated by stresses of various kinds in the body.

Vitamin E, besides being a powerful antioxidant and helpful in dealing with side effects (see "Dealing with Side Effects" in chapter 3), may protect against heart damage from the popular chemotherapy doxorubicin, as some animal studies have shown.

Books

Michael Lerner, Ph.D., *Choices in Healing: Integrating the Best of Conventional and Complementary Approaches to Cancer* (Cambridge, MA: MIT Press, 1994).

W. John Diamond, M.D., and W. Lee Cowden, M.D., with Burton Goldberg, *An Alternative Medicine Definitive Guide to Cancer* (Tiburon, CA: Future Medicine Publishing, 1997).

Organization

American Association of Naturopathic Physicians
601 Valley Street, Suite 105
Seattle, WA 98109
Phone: 206-298-0125
Website: www.naturopathic.org

A national list of physicians costs five dollars when ordered in hard copy, or you may view it on their website.

Supplier

L & H Vitamins
Phone: 800-221-1152

There are many vitamin supply houses; this company has good variety and prices.

Vitamins: Vitamin C

A controversial study by Nobel Prize winner Linus Pauling found life-extending results using vitamin C with terminal cancer patients. He placed one hundred people on 2 1/2 grams of powdered vitamin C four times a day and left one thousand patients with no vitamin therapy. The individuals on vitamin C lived significantly longer than those receiving no vitamin therapy. The Mayo Clinic was unable to replicate his results because, according to Pauling, of the way they conducted the research project. Other research since his study indicates that vitamin C can increase the effectiveness of radiation, decrease side effects, and help protect bone marrow, and that it seems to be a worthy complementary supplement. The vitamin is nontoxic and water soluble, so excesses are eliminated from the body very quickly.

Persons on a low-salt diet should use ascorbic acid crystals, not sodium ascorbate, and people with gastrointestinal difficulties or pH imbalance, who need to limit their acid intake, can take calcium or sodium ascorbate, or vitamin C in buffered form.

One potential drawback is the rebound effect. People taking large doses of vitamin C have had their vitamin C levels drop to below normal after they stop taking the vitamin. This is thought to leave people open to infection or renewed growth of their cancer. Gradually reducing the dosage over a week or two is recommended to avoid this effect.

Pauling never saw vitamin C therapy as a cure for cancer but regarded it rather as a supplemental therapy capable of extending life. Pauling recommended taking 6 to 18 grams of vitamin C daily, plus additional vitamins and minerals.

Even better results were achieved by Abram Hoffer, M.D., a well-known proponent of vitamin C and orthomolecular medicine, an approach that uses naturally occurring substances of the body in high-dose supplement form. He used even larger doses and added selenium and other vitamins and minerals. If you are interested in this therapy, the book by Pauling and Cameron contains comprehensive information and is available through the Linus Pauling Institute.

Books

Ewan Cameron and Linus Pauling, *Cancer and Vitamin C,* rev. ed. (Philadelphia, PA: Camino Books, 1993).

Abram Hoffer, M.D., and Linus Pauling, *Vitamin C and Cancer* (Kingston, Ontario: Quarry Press, forthcoming 1998).

Organization

Linus Pauling Institute of Science and Medicine
571 Weniger Hall
Oregon State University
Corvallis, OR 97331-6512
Phone: 541-737-5075
Fax: 541-737-5077
email: lpi@orst.edu
Website: www.osu.orst.edu/dept/lpi

The institute does not give advice or make treatment recommendations. It is instead a research-oriented resource for information and scientific reprints. The institute's critical response to a 1998 study out of the University of Leicester, England, suggesting that vitamin C might be harmful, can be viewed at their website.

Provider

Abram Hoffer, M.D., Ph.D.
2727 Quadra Street, Suite 3
Victoria, British Columbia
Canada V8T 4E5
Phone: 250-386-8756

Vitamins and Supplements: Quality Issues

The quality and potency of supplements and vitamins varies widely. Add to this the many unscrupulous supplement manufacturers, who use inferior quality supplements, fillers, and misleading labeling, and choosing supplements becomes even more difficult. Good companies will provide you, on request, with independent laboratory analysis of their product.

There may also be a lesson in irradiated foods for supplement and vitamin users. Irradiated foods do not compost or rot. In essence, they act as if they are dead substances. Some people consider this reason enough to assume that these foods probably are not as good as live, nonirradiated foods. Organic, or live, vitamins, as they are sometimes called, supposedly can be assimilated more easily by the body than their chemical counterparts, but they are also significantly more expensive.

Books

Karolyn Gazella, *Buyer—Be Wise!: The Consumer's Guide to Buying Quality Nutritional Supplements* (Green Bay, WI: IMPAKT Communications, 1998). Available from publisher at P.O. Box 12496, Green Bay, WI 54307.

James F. Balch, M.D., and Phyllis A. Balch, C.N.C., *Prescription for Nutritional Healing: A Practical A–Z Reference* (Garden City Park, NY: Avery Publishing Group, 1997). Does not offer information specifically for cancer but does contain valuable information on vitamins and supplements and includes a list of high-quality vitamin and supplement providers.

Chapter Resources

Books

W. John Diamond, M.D., and W. Lee Cowden, M.D., with Burton Goldberg, *An Alternative Medicine Definitive Guide to Cancer* (Tiburon, CA: Future Medicine Publishing, 1997). Reviews the more popular alternative therapies.

John Fink, *Third Opinion: An International Directory to Alternative Therapy Centers for the Treatment of Cancer and Other Degenerative Diseases* (Garden City Park, NY: Avery Publishing Group, 1997). Excellent directory of alternatives, educational resources, support groups, and information services. Includes guidelines for choosing a therapy.

Michael Lerner, Ph.D., *Choices in Healing: Integrating the Best of Conventional and Complementary Approaches to Cancer* (Cambridge, MA: MIT Press, 1994). Excellent, must-read book by founder of Commonweal; it is a scientific, levelheaded examination of conventional and alternative approaches, and is generously available for viewing in its entirety at Commonweal's website: www.commonwealhealth.org.

Ralph W. Moss, Ph.D., *Cancer Therapy: The Independent Consumer's Guide to Nontoxic Treatment and Prevention* (New York: Equinox Press, 1992). Excellent resource that gives short description of research on many therapies, including references and charts showing the effects of each on various cancers.

Ross Pelton, Ph.D., and Lee Overholser, Ph.D., *Alternatives in Cancer Therapy: The Complete Guide to Nontraditional Treatments* (New York: Simon & Schuster, 1994).

Richard Walters, *Options: The Alternative Cancer Therapy Book* (Garden City Park, NY: Avery Publishing Group, 1993). Reviews many popular alternative therapies.

Reports

Office of Alternative Medicine, *Alternative Medicine: Expanding Medical Horizons* (Washington, DC: Government Printing Office, 1994). Prepared for the National Institutes of Health. Although it has received little publicity, it is a good review of alternative treatments and recommendations for further study. Available for $25 from the Government Printing Office, phone: 202-512-1800, stock no. 017-040-00537-7.

Office of Technology Assessment, *Unconventional Cancer Treatments* (Washington, DC: Government Printing Office, 1990). Describes the unconventional treatments, legal and otherwise, most frequently used by cancer patients in the U.S. Available from the Government Printing Office, phone: 202-783-3238, report no. OTA-H-405

Research Services

For full descriptions of the following organizations, see the research services listed under "Choosing an Alternative Treatment" in chapter 4.

The Health Resource
564 Locust Street
Conway, AR 72032
Phone: 501-329-5272

Healing Choices
144 St. John's Place
Brooklyn, NY 11217
Phone: 718-636-4433

People Against Cancer
Alternative Therapy Program
604 East Street
P.O. Box 10
Otho, IA 50569-0010
Phone: 515-972-4444

World Research Foundation
41 Bell Rock Plaza, Suite C
Sedona, AZ 86351
Phone: 520-284-3300 or 1-818-999-5483

Organizations

Organizations that offer workshops or retreats to help people deal with cancer and/or choose a treatment program that is right for them are listed in Resources, section D. The following organizations provide information on alternative and supplemental therapies.

International Association of Cancer Victors and Friends
7740 West Manchester Avenue, #213
Playa del Rey, CA 90293
Phone: 310-822-5032

Foundation for Advancement of Cancer Therapies
P.O. Box 1242
Old Chelsea Station
New York, NY 10113
Phone: 212-741-2790

Center for Advancement in Cancer Education
300 East Lancaster Avenue, Suite 100
Wynnewood, PA 19096
Phone: 215-642-4810

Office of Alternative Medicine Clearinghouse
P.O. Box 8218
Silver Spring, MD 20907
Phone: 1-888-644-6226
Fax-back System: 800-531-1794
Website: altmed.od.nih.gov. (Choose "Research Grants," then "Grant
Award and Research Data," then "OAM Grants Database"; then type in
the search word *cancer.*)

University of Texas Center for Alternative Medicine Research in Cancer
P.O. Box 20186; #434
Houston, TX 77225
Website: www.sph.uth.tmc.edu/utcam/

National Foundation of Alternative Medicine
1155 Connecticut Avenue, N.W., Suite 300
Washington, DC 20036
Phone: 202-429-6633

An organization founded by Berkley Bedell (see interview in chapter 4)
that investigates alternative treatments for disease worldwide.

Part 3

Mind-Body Interventions

6

Mind-Body Therapies

For centuries, traditional medical systems from many cultures have appreciated and made use of the power of the mind to affect the body. The scientifically accepted "placebo effect" is probably the most well known proof of this ability. A placebo is an inactive substitute given as if it were a real dose of a needed drug. Placebos are used in drug research to compare the effects of a new drug to no treatment at all. The placebo effect is seen in the roughly one-third of patients who have at least some beneficial response to taking the placebo because they *believe* it is the medicine. In fact, before the advent of modern medicine, the placebo effect for centuries was a central treatment offered by physicians.

During the past thirty years, the growing body of research indicating connections between our minds and our bodies has shattered the long-held belief in Western medicine that these two systems were separate. The evidence is clear. The mind can have an effect on the quality of life and even on the course of an illness. The body of knowledge tracing the effects of our minds, thoughts, and emotions on health has come to be called mind-body medicine, and the techniques used are called mind-body interventions or therapies. These approaches are rapidly gaining acceptance in mainstream medicine as viable complementary therapies.

Some mind-body interventions are behavioral. They use physical or mental activities like meditation or imagery to influence the body, and they are discussed in this chapter. Psychology is another mind-body intervention that explores the relationship of a person's mental processes to disease; it is discussed in chapter 7.

One of the criticisms of some mind-body approaches, like imagery or psychological interventions, is that they can leave the patient feeling like a failure if the approach does not produce results. Patients need to help themselves by remembering that trying any therapy that doesn't work for you does not mean you are a failure, or incapable. Some approaches work for some people; some do not. It is important not to take it personally. Let it go, and move on. If you find you are being self-critical, remind yourself that your willingness to have tried only demonstrates your courage and your will to live.

Neuroimmunomodulation (NIM) and Psychoneuroimmunology (PNI)

In recent years, scientific exploration of the mind's ability to affect our bodies has begun in earnest. Neuroimmunomodulation (NIM) has become the most popular and promising area of research for immunologists and neuroscientists worldwide. *Neuro* refers to the nervous system, the brain, and the spinal cord. *Immuno* refers to the immune system, and *modulation* indicates that these systems interact and modulate, or change, each other.

According to Dr. Herbert Spector, a physiologist and scientist who is often referred to as the father of neuroimmunomodulation, you cannot stimulate one system without there being some reaction in the other systems. He says that the earliest experiments showing a psychological or behavioral influence on immunity were those of Serge Metalnikof, a scientist at the Pasteur Institute, in 1924. Metalnikof demonstrated that by using a Pavlovian type of conditioning he could change immune responses without the presence of a bacteria or virus. Since then, he and other scientists worldwide have conducted similar experiments proving that the mind does affect the immune system.

In these experiments, designed to test immune- and nervous-system interaction, nerve endings have been discovered in the tissues of the immune system. Changes in the brain and spinal cord have altered immune response. Immune-system cells can produce neurotransmitters that "talk" to the nervous system, and it responds, in turn, to neurotransmitters.

Psychoneuroimmunology (PNI) is a relatively new and closely related field of study. It examines how the mind, the nervous system, and the emotions all affect the immune system. Immune-system cells have been found to respond to stress hormones. It has also been demonstrated that stress makes the human immune system less responsive, and stress has also been shown to increase tumor growth in mice. Findings like these have provided hard evidence to support the potential for psychological interventions for the treatment of disease (see chapter 7). Experiments by PNI pioneer Dr. Robert Ader and others have led to the development of psycho-oncology, the study of psychological factors and their effects on cancer, and an increase in the use and study of various mind-body techniques as complementary cancer therapies.

Books

Steven E. Locke, M.D., and Douglas Colligan, *The Healer Within: The New Medicine of Mind and Body* (New York: New American Library, 1986).

Robert Ader, David L. Felton, and Nicolas Cohen, eds., *Psychoneuroimmunology*, 2d ed. (San Diego, CA: Academic Press, 1991).

Organization

Mind/Body Health Sciences, Inc.
393 Dixon Road
Boulder, CO 80302
Phone: 303-440-8460

This is the organization founded by Joan Borysenko, Ph.D., who was a pioneer in psychoneuroimmunology and cofounded the Mind/Body Clinic at the Harvard Medical School (see interview, below).

Meditation

Experiments in which animals have been subjected to some form of stress have demonstrated an increase in the rate of their tumor growth. Conversely, it is believed that by reducing stress, the immune system will be better able to fight cancer. Michael Lerner, Ph.D., in

Choices in Healing: Integrating the Best of Conventional and Complementary Approaches to Cancer (Cambridge, MA: MIT Press, 1994), discusses the work of Australian psychiatrist Ainslie Meares, who documented cases of cancer regression in clients who used meditation. Meares worked with seventy-three patients who participated in a minimum of twenty meditation sessions each. Lerner quotes Meares's findings:

> Nearly all such patients should expect significant reduction of anxiety and depression together with much less discomfort and pain. There is reason to expect a ten percent chance of quite remarkable slowing of the growth of the tumor, and a ten percent chance of less marked but still significant slowing. The results indicate that patients with advanced cancer have a ten percent chance of regression of the growth. There is a fifty percent chance of greatly improved quality of life, and for those who die, a ninety percent chance of death with dignity.

Meditation techniques vary, but all usually elicit a similar response, which has been dubbed the *relaxation response* by conventional medicine. The relaxation response is mainstream medicine's version of meditation, and has been popularized by Dr. Herbert Benson. Increasingly, relaxation is being used and taught at hospitals and clinics.

Dr. Joan Borysenko, cofounder of Harvard's Mind/Body Clinic, in her interview for the documentary *Cancer: Increasing Your Odds for Survival,* described several kinds of basic meditation techniques that are taught at the clinic (see interview, below). These include basic breathing techniques, such as focusing attention on breathing from the belly, which alter the input to and the response of the nervous system and elicit the relaxation response. To teach meditation as concentration, people are invited to think of a word or phrase and to let go of any other thoughts; this, too, elicits the relaxation response. Another meditation consists of learning to let thoughts come and go without becoming wrapped up in them.

For many people, just sitting still is difficult. Part of the value of meditating is becoming aware of your body and feelings. Andrew Weil, M.D., who has authored a popular and well-designed self-help wellness program, recommends in his book *8 Weeks to Optimum Health* (New York: Fawcett, 1998) meditating for five minutes a day and taking walks. These activities help people become aware of their bodies and feelings. He maintains that this is an important initial step to self-healing and to being able, eventually, to gain access to healing information from within (see "Internal Wisdom," chapter 8).

Finding a class in guided meditation is one good way to learn how to meditate. Many clinics offer in-depth training in meditation, and some offer meditation classes specifically used for pain management.

Books

Lawrence LeShan, Ph.D., *How to Meditate: A Guide to Self-Discovery* (New York: Bantam Books, 1984).

Stephen Levine, *A Gradual Awakening: An Introduction to Buddhist Meditation* (Garden City, NY: Anchor/Doubleday, 1979). An introduction to Buddhist meditation.

Stephen Levine, *Guided Meditations, Explorations, and Healings* (New York: Anchor/Doubleday, 1991). An excellent collection of guided meditations for a variety of purposes, including healing, pain, conscious dying, and grief.

Joan Borysenko, Ph.D., and Miroslav Borysenko, *The Power of the Mind to Heal* (Carson, CA: Hay House, 1994).

Thich Nhat Hanh, *Being Peace* (Berkeley, CA: Parallax Press, 1987).

Supplier

Simonton Cancer Center
P.O. Box 890
Pacific Palisades, CA 90272
Phone: 800-338-2360

Offers tapes and books on meditation.

Affirmations

Affirmations work on the theory, shared by mainstream psychology, that our beliefs play a large role in the kinds of possibilities we see and experience in our lives. The purpose of repeating affirmations is to help us replace old, limiting beliefs with newer, healthier ones.

Much of psychology is based on the reworking of our old beliefs. It is generally understood in psychology that our unconscious beliefs determine what kinds of possibilities we see in the world, attract, and ultimately manifest in our lives. Therapy is the process of replacing unhealthy beliefs with new, truer beliefs that can eventually attract a different set of physical circumstances.

For example, physically or psychologically abusive relationships can leave a child—let's say a girl—with the belief, "I am not worthy." As the child's' life progresses, she will focus on events she experienced that seem to agree with her belief of unworthiness and overlook those events that run counter to it. The idea behind affirmations is that simply repeating a new belief or affirmation, such as "I AM worthy," will allow the new belief to eventually replace the old, negative belief.

Experience has shown that repetition or affirmation of a mental belief can change the belief in the mind, but there is also a physical, emotional, energetic remembrance of the event/belief that is stored in the body. Unless the emotional component of the old belief is also released from the body it will slowly keep repeating its message and gradually reestablish the belief on the mental level. That is why most people need professional support and therapies that also address the way the belief is stored in the body and emotions to achieve more permanent results.

Some books give one-affirmation-fits-all statements for many different health and emotional problems, just as some dream interpretation books offer generic interpretations of dream symbols. Psychologists understand that generic dream interpretations usually do not speak to the individual's unique psyche. Competent psychotherapists understand that the only reliable and accurate associations are those derived from the client's own explorations, where the client determines her or his own meaning for or association with a dream or an event.

Client-specific applications are also needed when it comes to affirmations. For example, to say that all back problems are caused by someone's issues about feeling a lack of support, and to prescribe one affirmation for all back problems, is simplistic. While the affirmation may help some, it will have little effect for others.

Someone who has the ability, through meditation and self-awareness, to accurately assess their own self-limiting beliefs and who can construct appropriate affirmations that challenge those beliefs, can use affirmations without assistance. However, this skill is rare. A counselor or therapist familiar with this "mind technology" is probably the best route to go to help create individual affirmations that are most deeply effective.

Books

Louise Hay, *You Can Heal Your Life* (Santa Monica, CA: Hay House, 1984).

Paramahansa Yogananda, *Scientific Healing Affirmations* (Los Angeles, CA: Self-Realization Fellowship, 1998).

Imagery

According to Jeanne Achterberg, author of *Imagery in Healing* (Boston, MA: Shambhala Publications, 1985), "Imagery is the thought process that invokes and uses the senses. . . . It is the communication mechanism between perception, emotion and bodily change." In some Eastern thought it is said that we can do nothing, not even a simple movement, without first developing an image for it. There are two basic types of healing imagery: receptive and active. Receptive imagery is using a quiet meditative state to receive inner information (see "Internal Wisdom," chapter 8). Active imagery is actively visualizing some desired result.

Active imagery includes two kinds of imagery techniques: process imagery and end-state imagery. Process imagery is actively visualizing, in scientific detail, the healing process for your specific cancer. You use process imagery when you have researched the medical processes involved in the healing you need and very specifically see the medicine or immune system working with the problem that causes your illness.

End-state, or goal-oriented, imagery is when you visualize the desired end-state of health. You may see white light, God, or whatever your image of a healing force is, and you trust the inner healing force to do whatever is necessary to reach that state of health you are visualizing.

Susan Sperry, M.S.N., was the lead therapist at the Exceptional Cancer Patients Program, where she used a variety of techniques, including imagery, in working with cancer patients. In my documentary *Cancer: Increasing Your Odds For Survival,* she suggested that process imagery should not be used when you are feeling weak but should be saved, instead, for when you are feeling strong:

> If you're not feeling strong, you don't want to do an imagery where you're bringing in an image of your cancer. Because you're likely to empower the cancer, because you're not feeling strong yourself. When you're feeling weak or frightened, it's much more important for you to do an image of just general, overall well-being. Then when you feel stronger, you can do something where you visualize your immune system really dealing with this cancer in a very effective way.

Some experts on imagery suggest that process imagery is more effective in curing illness, which makes sense if it is specifically tailored to you. A possible course of action would then be to use receptive imagery first, listening for helpful inner healing information, and then developing a personalized healing image. To do this, most people need the help of a therapist, social worker, or counselor who is skilled in this type of exploration. Broad or generic healing images may or may not be helpful. Hitting the nail on the head with individually tailored imagery will be more effective.

One example of receptive imagery, recommended by Achterberg, looks like this: You might meditate, becoming relaxed and going deep within for about ten minutes, and then you look at and face the problem, illness, or pain. (This differs from many visualization efforts that avoid contact with the source of the problem.) Then, try being receptive to the sights, sounds, smells, and feelings of the problem, at least for a few minutes, especially in your first sessions, until you develop some understanding, knowledge of, and image for it. Then see your inner healing force gathering around the edges of the problem and then entering and facilitating whatever learning or healing process you are undertaking.

Proponents of the use of imagery disagree on which kind is helpful for which illnesses. Some say the imagery has to be different for immune as opposed to autoimmune diseases and that using the wrong one could be counterproductive. Others say that relying on the inner healing wisdom will avoid any unproductive efforts.

If you want to use imagery, it's clear that:

- You have to believe that the imagery can help you to heal; otherwise it will not.

- You must be willing to invest time and effort. (Achterberg recommends twenty minutes per session—ten to go deep within yourself and ten devoted to imagery.)

- You need to read up on the subject, listen to tapes, and, preferably, employ professional guidance.

- You must not expect to visualize like you are watching a movie. Rarely does anyone see bright, distinct images. Usually people just see a form or feel a sense of something present; such images are adequate.

- You need to ask yourself if this feels right for you and if you should pursue it. If not, don't bother with it. Use your time to pursue those things that intuitively feel correct for you.

Imagery is a subtle and potentially powerful technique, but it must be learned well, and it requires discipline to practice. Following a guided imagery led by a voice on an audiotape or by someone in person is an excellent way to start learning how to do meditation and imagery (see "Simonton Approach," chapter 7).

Books

Jeanne Achterberg, Ph.D., *Imagery in Healing: Shamanism and Modern Medicine* (Boston, MA: Shambhala Publications, 1985).

Errol R. Korn and Karen Johnson, *Visualization: The Uses of Imagery in the Health Professions* (Homewood, IL: Dow Jones-Irwin, 1983).

Martin Rossman, M.D., *Healing Yourself: A Step-by-Step Program for Better Health Through Imagery* (New York: Walker, 1987).

Stephen Levine, *Healing into Life and Death* (New York: Anchor/Doubleday, 1987).

Organizations

Simonton Cancer Center
P.O. Box 890
Pacific Palisades, CA 90272
Phone: 800-338-2360

Offers tapes and publications.

Warm Rock Tapes
P.O. Box 100
Chamisal, NM 87525
Phone: 800-731-HEAL

Offers tapes and publications.

Academy for Guided Imagery
P.O. Box 2070
Mill Valley, CA 94942
Phone: 800-726-2070

Offers publications, tapes, and a directory of practitioners trained in guided imagery.

Music Therapy

Music has been used to aid healing throughout history. The philosopher and mathematician Pythagoras taught his students to change the emotional states of fear, sorrow, worry, and anger through singing and playing a musical instrument. The effects of music on breathing, blood pressure, digestion, and muscular activity were first documented during the Renaissance. Music therapy had its professional debut in America after World War II when the Veterans Administration Hospital began using music to help rehabilitate returning soldiers.

More recently, new-age practitioners have developed sound-oriented therapies, including "toning." Toning, not unlike shamanistic singing among native medicine people, consists of the practitioner or the patient making distinct sounds or tones directed at specific areas of illness, energetic blockages, or chakras. Chakras in Eastern energy medicine are energy centers in the body that correspond to specific body systems, organs, and glands. These tones are meant to create vibrations that bring energetic healing to the organism. Some musicians are producing recordings specifically designed to stimulate and balance these chakras to promote healing and to enhance states of consciousness.

Western medical research has established the usefulness of music in many areas, including as a pain reliever, as a relaxant and anxiety reducer for infants and children, and as a method for facilitating communication with terminally ill individuals about their feelings and disease. A 1985 study demonstrated that music could suppress stress hormones in orthopedic, gynecologic, and urologic patients.

Relaxation and imagery are also assisted by listening to music.

Music can facilitate self- or therapist-guided imagery and is used to lessen anxieties and fears associated with hospitalization and dying. Some have found that music therapy lessens nausea and vomiting during and following chemotherapy.

If you are interested in music therapy as a complementary therapy, ask at the hospital if they have a music therapy program, or contact the American Music Therapy Association for music therapists in your area. If you are going to be in the hospital or will be spending time receiving unpleasant or stressful treatments, you may wish to take a portable tape player with you. Bring your favorite music, and consider asking your friends to bring you tapes.

Book

Deforia Lane, Ph.D., MT-B, *Music as Medicine: Deforia Lane's Life of Music, Healing and Faith* (Grand Rapids, MI: Zondervan, 1995).

Organization

American Music Therapy Association
8455 Colesville Road, Suite 1000
Silver Spring, MD 20910
Phone: 301-589-3300

Provides free information and referrals.

Humor

Laughter has a multitude of beneficial effects on the body. It is effective in pain management and improves immune function. Having a fun-filled life works to this end as well. As an adjunct therapy, what could be better?

Norman Cousins is best known for attributing his healing to laughter. He developed ankylosing spondylitis, a progressive spinal disorder, and was told that he had less than a one-in-five-hundred chance of recovering. Cousins reasoned that if negative thinking could make you sick, then positive thinking should make you better. He checked himself out of the hospital and checked himself into a hotel room, where he proceeded to medicate himself with Marx

Brothers movies, *Candid Camera* shows, and other things that made him laugh. He found that for every ten minutes of laughter, he was able to get two hours of pain-free, uninterrupted sleep—which was remarkable for this very painful disease. He not only recovered from ankylosing spondylitis, he also became an adjunct professor of medicine at the UCLA medical school, and lectured and wrote extensively about mind-and-body medicine.

Books

Norman Cousins, *Anatomy of an Illness as Perceived by the Patient* (New York: Bantam, 1981).

Norman Cousins, *Head First: The Biology of Hope and the Healing Power of the Human Spirit* (New York: Penguin, 1990).

Joyce Saltman, Ph.D., Ed.D., *Sing a Celebration* (Watertown, MA: Ivory Tower, 1988). A collection of funny lyrics to well-known songs, designed to lift the spirit.

Video and Audio tape

Laughter: Rx for Survival is a video and audiotape of a talk given by Joyce Saltman, an international lecturer on the topic of humor and healing. Available from:

Mirth Works
30 Lenox Avenue
Norwalk, CT 06854
Phone: (203) 853-8002

Practitioner

Joyce Saltman
Phone: 203-272-9519

Organization

The HUMOR Project
480 Broadway, Suite 210
Saratoga Springs, NY 12866
Phone: 518-587-8770

Hypnosis

Unlike theatrical hypnosis, clinical or therapeutic hypnosis does not involve losing awareness of everyday reality. It is usually a light trance state where clients are aware of what is happening around them and they maintain voluntary control. It is very similar to guided meditation. It can be used like receptive imagery to gather information, or like active imagery to try and enhance wellness or immunity. Skilled practitioners of hypnosis can help clients replace dysfunctional beliefs with new, healthier beliefs on a subconscious level. My own belief is that hypnosis can be helpful, but it depends on the skill of the therapist. If the idea of hypnosis as a way of helping to change beliefs appeals to you, I suggest pursuing it only if you have a competent therapist with whom you are comfortable.

Books

Stephen C. Parkhill, *Answer Cancer: Miraculous Healings Explained: The Healing of a Nation* (Deerfield Beach, FL: Health Communications, 1995).

Ernest Rossi, *The Psychobiology of Mind/Body Healing: New Concepts of Therapeutic Hypnosis,* rev. ed. (New York: W. W. Norton, 1993). More for professionals, but a scholarly resource for those interested in the science of hypnosis.

Michael Lerner, Ph.D., *Choices in Healing: Integrating the Best of Conventional and Complementary Approaches to Cancer* (Cambridge, MA: MIT Press, 1994). Includes excellent overview of hypnosis in chapter 10. Can be viewed at the Commonweal website: www.commonwealhealth.org.

Organizations

American Society of Clinical Hypnosis
2200 East Devon Avenue, Suite 291
Des Plaines, IL 60018
Phone: 847-297-3317

Society for Clinical and Experimental Hypnosis (SCEH)
2201 Haeder Road, Suite 1
Pullman, WA 99163
Phone: 509-332-7555
Fax: 509-332-5907
E-mail: sceh@pullman.com
Website: sunsite.utk.edu/IJCEH/scehframe.htm

Interview with
Joan Borysenko, Ph.D.

on Psychoneuroimmunology and Bodymind, Prayer and Psychotherapy, the Changing Face of Medicine, and the Inner Healer

Dr. Joan Borysenko is a cancer cell biologist, a licensed psychologist, and an authority on mind-body medicine. She cofounded the Mind/Body Clinic at the Beth Israel Hospital, which moved later to the New England Deaconess Hospital, one of Harvard's teaching hospitals, and she is a former instructor in medicine at Harvard Medical School. She was a pioneer in the medical synthesis called psychoneuroimmunology. As stated in the title of the book she recently cowrote with her husband, Dr. Borysenko believes in the power of the mind to heal. She wrote the *New York Times* best-seller *Minding the Body, Mending the Mind,* and also *Fire in the Soul: A New Psychology of Spiritual Optimism; Guilt Is the Teacher, Love Is the Lesson;* and *On Wings of Light: Meditations for Awakening to the Source.* She resides in Colorado, where she founded the organization Mind/Body Health Sciences (see "Neuroimmunomodulation and Psychoneuroimmunology," above). She is a gracious person who is able to explain complex and esoteric subjects in accessible, human terms.

You began your academic career pursuing a doctoral degree in cellular biology. What then caused you to become interested in the effects the mind has on the body?

I was originally a tumor cell biologist working in the laboratory growing cancer cells. My interests had narrowed down to which molecules in the cancer cell surface caused cancer cells to become antisocial—to go other places in the body and to finally become destructive. I didn't know anything about a *whole person* who had cancer.

When my own father developed leukemia and finally died—not actually of the leukemia but from side effects of medication—I realized I did not want to work with isolated cells anymore; I wanted to work with whole human beings who had cancer. That led me to change my career. I left the laboratory as a tumor cell biologist and took a second postdoctoral fellowship—a National Institutes of Health Fellowship—at Harvard Medical School with Dr. Herbert Benson and retrained in behavioral medicine.

You mentioned in one of your books that research suggests that the body and mind are not separate entities but are actually one, which you call body-mind. Can you explain what that is and tell us what convinced you of that?

It is remarkable to me that any of us could have forgotten that we have one body-mind and not a mind *and* a body. Who is there who hasn't had a really embarrassing thought and then instantly blushed and recognized—of course, I have one body-mind! A thought or emotion causes my entire vasculature system to change, my entire hormonal profile to change. Now we know that's true. Our very thoughts and emotions affect the hormonal profile in our blood. They affect our heart rate and may affect our immune system.

Was it those kind of experiences that made you believe that the body-mind was one entity, or did you come around to it more from your research?

The two most fascinating instances, for me, [of insight] into how the body and mind [co]exist were diametrically opposed. One was an experience when I was a child of six, and the other was [reading] a research publication that I found years later when I was a scientist. As a six-year-old, I had an uncle who despised cheese. Lots of people hate certain foods so much that they will throw up even at the thought of them. This is what happened to him. He ate a piece of cheesecake at our house, didn't recognize it for what it was, and an hour later when my mother said, "Hey Dick, I thought you hated cheese!" I watched this beautiful man throw up on the rug in front of me. It was clear to me that it was not a physiological effect of the cheese, but that something in his *mind* caused this tremendous upheaval in his body.

What caught my mind as a research scientist was a report by Dr. Robert Ader about a psychoneuroimmunology experiment. Psychoneuroimmunology is the study of how our emotional state affects our nervous system and how those in combination affect our immune system. The experiment was about conditioning in the rat. We all know about classical conditioning—Pavlov paired meat powder with a bell, and when he would ring the bell the dog would salivate. Well, Ader did that with rats and their immune function. He paired a funny taste, in this case saccharin or apple juice and water, with the administration of a drug that suppressed the immune system. Later, if he just gave rats the funny-tasting water, they would automatically suppress their immune systems. When I realized that you could classically condition immunological function, I said, "Hey! We've got something really neat to look at here!"

How do you define psychoneuroimmunology?

Psychoneuroimmunology is made up of three terms: *psycho*, which has to do with mind, thoughts, emotions; *neuro*, which has to do with the nervous system; and *immunology*, having to do with the immune system. It studies the effects of our thoughts and emotions on our body's susceptibility or resistance to disease.

This field began a long time ago, maybe in the 1930s, with the research of Dr. Hans Selye, the "Father of Stress." He found that if you chronically stressed animals, then certain changes occurred in their bodily organs—notably, the adrenal glands, which release stress hormones, got bigger and bigger and bigger. Also, their thymus glands, one of the prime glands that has to do with lymphocyte function—lymphocytes being white blood cells of the immune system—the thymus gland got involuted or shrunken under chronic stress. This was the first indication that stress and the immune system had something to do with one another.

About twenty years ago, Dr. Robert Ader at the University of Rochester began an interesting series of experiments: for example, if rats were handled as babies, they had more resistance to disease than rats who were not handled as babies. In recent years, Ader and many others have begun to look at both the neurological and the hormonal impact of stress on the immune system.

Has a two-way communication system between the mind and the immune system been discovered?

Yes, a two-way system of communication has been well established between the brain and the immune system. For example, when antibodies are being produced by the immune system, you can actually record in one of the ventramedial nuclei of the hypothalamus of the brain an increase in the amount of electrical stimulation. Clearly, the brain knows when the immune system is functioning; and, by the same token, if you stimulate different areas of the brain, you can preferentially cause certain changes in the immune system—both suppression of the immune system and enhancement of the immune system.

Another part of that two-way street is neuropeptides (very small proteins). We used to think that the brain was primarily a switching station. Now we know that it is the largest *gland* in the body: it *puts out* over sixty of these neuropeptides. The neuropeptides are produced primarily in the part of the brain known as the *limbic system*, the system where we process our emotions. It seems that each one of our emotions has a neuropeptide "fingerprint," and when we feel an emotion, the large gland called the brain lets go of these neuropeptides, for which we have receptors on every cell of our immune system. By the same token, the cells of the immune system also secrete neuropeptides, which can come back up to stimulate the brain. So, this idea that the brain is somehow protected from hormonal input from the rest of the body doesn't seem true anymore; we know we have a communication that goes in both directions.

What is the Mind-Body Clinic, and what does the program consist of?

In 1981 I cofounded a mind-body clinic at one of the Harvard teaching hospitals, along with Dr. Herbert Benson and a psychiatrist, Dr. Ilan Kutz. We taught patients ways to use their minds to benefit their physical bodies. Dr. Herbert Benson is noted for his research in the relaxation response, an innate physiological response and the counterpart of the body stress, or "fight or flight" response. Whenever a person goes into a state of focused attention, for example during a meditative exercise or relaxation procedure, they bring forth this integrated hypothalamic response. Heart rate goes down, blood pressure goes down, and there are certain beneficial hormonal alterations. The actual brain wave pattern changes. In addition to that, recent research has indicated that the relaxation response can improve immunological function, in the cases where that function has been depressed—by the aging process, for example. We tried in the mind-body clinic to teach these researched kinds of changes to patients so that, along with whatever Western physical medicine they needed for their condition, they could also learn to use their minds beneficially.

How accepted is psychoneuroimmunology by other hospitals and mainstream medical professions?

Research in the field of psychoneuroimmunology has given much more credibility to the mind-body interaction. Nowadays people often refer to all mind-body interactions as psychoneuroimmunology. But psychoneuroimmunology, or PNI as it is often called, is only one part of a much larger interaction between mind and body. I think that the whole mind-body field, including psychoneuroimmunology, is slowly gaining ground in hospital practice.

At the Mind-Body Clinic, what were the types of relaxation techniques that you taught, and what results did you obtain?

We taught people a variety of ways to bring forth the relaxation response. We taught simple breathing techniques. Most people are aware that when you breathe from your belly the body tends to relax, [for one reason] because you are concentrating your focus of attention on belly breathing, and this elicits the relaxation response. It is basically a simple form of *meditation*, the focusing of attention.

We also taught simple forms of concentration and meditation: the person thinks of a word or phrase—secular or nonsecular—focuses on that, and lets go of extraneous thoughts when they come. Again, they will elicit the relaxation response. We also taught different forms of meditation, one called *mindfulness*, which is simply learning to let thoughts come and go without becoming wrapped up in the them; just let them be. We also taught techniques of creative imagination and problem solving—things that help people cope with having a physical illness.

What were the results of participating in the program?

Results for most people fell into two categories. One was that most people felt better psychologically; they were less anxious, less depressed, less helpless. They felt much more in control of their lives, depending on the physical difficulty that brought them in.

We have to remember that 75 to 80 percent of the time people visit their family doctors for stress-related disorders. In a majority of instances these disorders will disappear completely. I am talking here about various gastrointestinal complaints, headaches, back pain. Very often headaches, even migraines, have a large stress component. These disappear entirely or are significantly ameliorated [through relaxation techniques]. Even things like insulin-dependent diabetes: you can't eliminate diabetes with these techniques, but research shows that, because stress hormones increase your need for blood sugar, people with diabetes who practice these relaxation techniques actually require less insulin and have fewer incidences of either high or low blood sugar; it tends to stabilize their metabolism to some degree.

When we get to things like cancer, you really need to have a research protocol of the sort that we did not have. As you know, there are always people with cancer who do much better than their prognoses would have suggested, and I have certainly had many patients like that; but there we are primarily looking at the clinic's enhancement of *quality* of life, not *quantity* of life.

Your second book Guilt Is the Teacher, Love Is the Lesson *is about far more than guilt. How would you describe the book?*

It had to do with observations I made while at the Mind-Body Clinic. I left the clinic in 1988, and I began to wonder what the common denominator was that people there were trying to learn. What was it that makes us susceptible to stress and erodes the quality of life? I began to recognize that it was the sense of worthlessness that many people have, and I began to think about how that came up for people, particularly people who would come to see me with life-threatening illnesses. [These people] would usually ask, "Why me? Why did this happen to me?"

I found that people answered that question in many different ways. Some said, "I really don't know why" or "Maybe it was some lifestyle difficulty that I had—I smoked—but whatever it is, I am going to pick up my life and do the best that I can." I found that there were also people who would answer in a very guilty kind of way, saying, "Because I am not good enough; I have done something wrong." Beyond simple psychological self-blame, I found that a number of people also brought God into the picture. They would say, "This bad thing is happening to me because I am being punished for my sins." This surprised me. As a psychologist, I have been taught that religion is something that we don't get into; and yet, I found that most people have a real strong idea of what a higher power is for them. Very often this idea is some leftover from childhood religious teachings. Sometimes it is a beautiful idea that gives them self-esteem and helps them live their life in a kind and loving manner. But sometimes their idea of God is like a punitive bogeyman, a petty Santa Claus looking over your shoulder to see whether or not you deserve toys. I recognized that as somebody who worked with people who had physical illnesses, and who also worked with people in psychotherapy, I needed to become much more aware of both the religious and spiritual dimensions of life, because these so clearly affected the process of healing.

A colleague of mine, an internist, Dr. Larry Dossey, has written several books, including *Recovering the Soul,* which I think is a wonderful title coming from a physician because it finally reminds us that it is not possible to look at medicine, psychology, and spirituality as separate disciplines. [Dossey] looks at the history of medicine in the West over the last one hundred years, dividing it into three eras. The first era has to do with the advent of the wonderful understanding of the cause and effect of disease. Sometimes it is hard to realize that it was only in World War II that we developed antibiotics; before that there wasn't much you could do about infection. And it was only in the 1920s that we found that vitamin C prevented scurvy.

So, in the last one hundred years we have gotten some very specific "magic bullets" that help with the variety of diseases. And surgical techniques have really improved. That is "Era I medicine." It is wonderful medicine, based on cause and effect and on knowing specific pathophysiological mechanisms that cause disease. However, it is not the whole picture.

I know I was very ill as a graduate student at Harvard Medical School, and I had every stress-related disorder known to humankind. In six months I had developed high blood pressure, migraine headaches, irritable bowel syndrome, dizzy spells, fainting spells, and an immune dysfunction that kept me hospitalized with pneumonia, chronic bronchitis, and pleurisy. I went to one of the best doctors that Harvard had, but for me the cure didn't lie in pills; it depended on learning what it was that created such internal stress that my whole mind-body went into an uproar. I said that 75 to 80 percent of all reasons why people visit the physician are for these mind-body disorders. So Dossey sees "Era II medicine" as the advent of mind-body medicine.

Now, mind-body and Era I, physical, medicine are both based on the same underlying premise. Here is something very important: that premise is that your mind—your consciousness—is a local biochemical phenomenon of your brain. By that I mean that you have synapses: certain biochemical things happen, and you transfer information from neuron to neuron, and that is what your consciousness is. The natural corollary, upon which all modern science is based, is that when you die, your brain dies. You lose your consciousness—that's the end. So [modern science] has no place in it for the soul. It has always been split off. It is like it is something else, not part of medicine.

Dossey's premise is that perhaps the soul *is* part of medicine. To him, Era III medicine has to do with the premise (which physicists tell us is quite likely) that [the] mind is nonlocal. It is not a simple epiphenomenon of nervous activity of *my* brain and *your* brain. It was Einstein who once said that the illusion that we are isolated is really an "optical delusion" of our consciousness. The physicist Schrödinger, who invented the wave equations of quantum mechanics, likewise said that if we could measure the sum total of the number of minds in the universe, there would in fact be just one. This means that some of the things that human beings have experienced all of their lives and that science has pooh-poohed need to be looked at once again.

For example, the National Opinion Research Council at the University of Chicago polled Americans in the 1970s and then again in the 1980s on common paranormal experiences. I do not like that word: I think they are really quite normal experiences, but things that really are based on this thought that consciousness might be shared. Five percent of the American public—that's eight million people—have had near-death experiences. It is hard to open a magazine these days without seeing some report of a near-death experience. This changed me as a medical scientist and a psychologist. I had patients who came to me and said, "I had a near-death experience" and would describe a sequence of lifting out of their bodies, looking down and seeing their bodies, and then moving through a tunnel. And then about 50 percent of them would talk about coming out into the presence of the light—described just as the mystics did, whether Christian, Buddhist, or Hindu. These patients say things like "the light is unknowable," but when pressed to describe it they will use words like *all-loving, all-forgiving, all-wisdom*—that in the presence of the light they recognized their own inner purity and their part in the divine plan.

That poll at the National Opinion Research Council also indicated that 67 percent of all Americans have said that they have been in contact with dead loved ones at some point. Over 50 percent have had experiences of ESP, knowing things that their physical senses could not have told them. About one-third of Americans say that they have been lifted out of themselves and have had some transcendent experience. When you measure these people in terms of mental health, interestingly, they score at the top of the scale for mental adjustment. So we are not talking about a few crackpots with weird experiences. We are talking about the most functional people in our society, and these people turn out to be very loving and down-to-earth people.

Now, how does this relate to medicine? Dossey says Era III medicine takes into account this idea that mind is not just a function of the brain but is nonlocal. Somehow it is all connected in a way that perhaps the physicists understand and that the mystics have experienced—and perhaps this can affect the physical body. He cites a number of fascinating studies that have been done on things like prayer.

One of the studies on prayer, published in 1988 in a Southern medical journal, got a great deal of press. It was conducted by a cardiologist, Dr. Randolph Byrd. Many physicians and therapists have heard reports from patients of things like the effect of prayer or out-of-body experiences or near-death experiences, and often doctors tuck those under the rug or say the patient is crazy. Byrd said, "Why not look at it scientifically? Let's see if prayer might have an effect." So he designed the gold standard of scientific studies—the randomized, double-blind study. He took four hundred patients admitted to the coronary intensive care unit at San Francisco General Hospital, and he randomized them into two groups. One group got the usual coronary intensive care; the other got the usual care, plus they were prayed for at a distance by prayer groups across the country who were given lists of names.

It was important that this study be double-blind. This means that neither the patient nor the staff knew who was being prayed for and who wasn't. This was important for two reasons. Number one, it ruled out the placebo effect, that if you thought prayer was good for you and you knew people were praying for you, there would be a chance you'd get better just because of that belief. That is a very important mind-body phenomenon in and of itself. Number two, it ruled out the Hawthorne effect, which is that whenever another person pays attention to us, we feel better. So if the staff believed in prayer and treated preferentially the people who were being prayed for—or, on the other hand, if the staff didn't believe in prayer and ignored those people—you would [risk] the Hawthorne effect. So the Hawthorne effect, too, was ruled out.

When the code was broken on the study, fascinating results occurred. The people that were prayed for did significantly better: fewer cardiac arrests, fewer cases of pulmonary edema, which is a potentially life-threatening accumulation of fluid in the lungs. There were fewer cases of infection and less need for antibiotics. The skeptics moved in to look at the study, which is a good thing. And no one is really able to fault the study; it is statistically sound.

My patients would often tell me things like, "I walked into the doctor's office, and after talking to him for two minutes I could feel that he was either a healing person or he felt toxic to me." Perhaps it has to do with what the doctor is sending out in his or her mind to the patient. Are they seeing this patient as whole person? Are they seeing the greatest potential for healing this person? Or, on the other hand, are they hurried or seeing the person as a statistic? I think most people know what a healing presence feels like, and what a non-healing presence feels like, and yet we have been told to ignore these things. Well, I am beginning to think they *do* make a difference. That's why it is so important for each of us to have a doctor that we can trust, someone who can practice the best in Era I physical medicine, a doctor who can support us in our use of mind-body medicine,

to initially is perfect for you, and it might be that it is step one in the long search. It has been said before that people spend much more time researching their next car than the doctor with whom they are going to have a long and healing relationship. The way that that doctor acts, not only the way they practice medicine from a technical aspect, but the way they act toward you—whether they can help you to be hopeful and maintain a sense that you can fight this, and whether when the time comes, they can also help you die—these are questions that you need to be able to ask the doctor in an outright way *and* also intuit about that person. And that often takes the help of friends.

After obtaining your support system and a good doctor, what are the most important things cancer patients should be doing if they want to survive?

First of all, you want to take the best possible care of your physical body that you can. Within whatever your appropriate limits are, exercise and eat right. There is a lot out there about diet and cancer, and to the best of my knowledge the best diet is high in fiber and fruits and vegetables and has minimum fats. Take care of those obvious bits of housekeeping. Make sure that you can get enough rest. In addition, I recommend finding some kind of program of relaxation, of stress reduction.

I think it is also important for people to finish unfinished business. Often it is when we get a life-threatening illness that we are motivated to do that. We ask ourselves, "Whom do I really need to forgive?" There are a lot of us who would like to hang on to regrets and resentments forever. Plenty of people are busy hating others who are long since dead. What you have to realize is that forgiveness is essentially something that you do for yourself. It sets the forgiver free. This is a very important thing to do because it takes a lot of mental energy to hold onto anger.

The other thing that is really important are support groups. We have research data from Dr. David Spiegal at Stanford. He had over fifty women with metastatic breast cancer whom he split into two groups. One got normal medical care, and the other [also] got a once-a-week support group for one year. The women in the support group lived twice as long as the women who got just medical care and no support group. At the end of ten years, even though they had begun with metastatic cancer, three of those women are still alive. These women would tell you it's not just for the quantity of life that support is important: To be with other people in crisis and to find the good in that situation—perhaps that is what healing is really about.

What makes you believe there is a universal self that is loving and wise and is the core of each person?

You can look at this from the experiences of ordinary people, from the experiences of saints and mystics, and from the very interesting research realm of psychopathology. Sometimes we learn more by studying the mind when it doesn't work properly than we ever could from studying the mind when it's whole. People with multiple personality disorder have been intensively studied. Usually this disorder begins when the person is severely abused as a child and basically dissociates from the situation of abuse and forms a totally separate personality. You might have a child who develops one personality to take care of siblings, another to take abuse, another to study. It is common for there to be two dozen different personalities. In the early 1970s a psychotherapist by the name of Ralph Allison found that when he hypnotized people with this disorder, he could regress them and find out the moment of abuse during which a certain personality split and formed. And then he found a fascinating thing—that within each person who had multiple personality disorder there was one personality that always claimed not to have been formed at a specific moment like all the rest. Regardless of the religious background of the person involved, that personality would describe itself with terms like "I am the wisdom self" or "I am a conduit for divine love" or "I am the divine spark of the person." Often this inner self would say things like "I have been with the person from the time before they took a body, and I will continue to be with that person until they lay their body down."

Interestingly enough, when Allison could communicate with this "inner-self helper," it would give very specific feedback about the therapy and the integration of all of those disparate subpersonalities or false selves into a functional whole. And because it was such a good therapeutic ally and had such reliable information, he came to call it the inner-self helper.

I think we are all a little bit like multiple personalities in that the work of a lifetime for each one of us is to let down those false selves and to come back in touch with the most true core of our being, which, to me, would be that inner-self helper. Some people might call it their intuition, some might call it a higher self, some a divine spark, some a soul—I think they are all talking about the same thing.

Would you please tell the story of Sally dying?

One of the first people that I ever had the privilege to sit with as they were dying was a young physician named Sally. She believed that consciousness was a function of the brain and that when she died, that would be the end of her consciousness. Well, I sat with her as she was dying—and many people who are dying kind of float out of consciousness and come back—and I asked her where she was when she had floated out, and she looked at me and started to laugh. She said that she had been completely wrong, and she described that she floated out of her body, seen us down below, floated through the wall, seen her record at the nursing station, and read her chart. She became aware of her parents outside the hospital coming in and noticed them going to the cafeteria and having lunch. As I am a skeptic by nature, I asked the parents later what they had for lunch, and it was just what Sally had described. She went on for the rest of that day to describe several predeath visions, which we know now are very common in people who are dying. The most beautiful part of this was that she came back and told me that on the other side there was a light. She told me about the tremendous sense of love and peace and beauty and the magnificence of that light and the magnificence of the human soul.

Here I had gone to console her in her time of dying, and she ended up consoling me. That is one of the experiences, for me, that stay there for a lifetime and that encourage me in moments when I identify with one my own false selves, forgetting that core of love and peace and beauty, a spark of which resides in our own heart as our most true identity.

[All interviews have been edited for length and clarity.]

Dr. Joan Borysenko lives in Colorado and lectures internationally. She may be reached through her organization:

Mind/Body Health Sciences Inc.
393 Dixon Road
Boulder, CO 80302
Phone: 303-440-8460

7

Psychological Aspects of Cancer

The connection between the mind and the body is nothing new to those involved in the practice and process of psychology. Psychosomatic medicine has long been a specialty in psychiatry. As we saw in the last chapter, psychoneuroimmunology (PNI) is a complementary area of study that specifically examines how psychological factors like thoughts, emotions, and stress affect our immune system and our susceptibility or resistance to disease. The existing body of knowledge in the field of psychology as it relates to disease, supported by PNI research, has spurred interest in psycho-oncology, the study of psychological factors and their effects on cancer.

Stress has been the subject of much of the research in these fields of study. Stress, a term that covers a variety of emotional states, has been proven to adversely affect the immune system. Chronic repressed emotions and chronic stress can reduce immune function, making a person more susceptible to diseases, including cancer. In body-oriented psychotherapies it is understood that the experience of emotions can be avoided or altered by tensing the body. In the Eastern medical model, this can result in a blockage in the natural flow of energy within the body, which is believed to be a precursor to disease. If this is true, psychotherapy may be a critical intervention for people whose emotional and psychological blocks may have stressed their immune systems or created such blockages. Psychotherapy can clear the mind and relieve emotions, preparing the body to be receptive to healing.

It is also possible that a person may have a belief embedded in their subconscious that impedes healing. For example, a person may have a belief she or he is not worthy of the positive things that life has to offer. On an unconscious level, they may not feel worthy of healing. In this situation the various forms of physical intervention may be falling on infertile ground. They could be treating the symptoms but not addressing issues that could have a direct impact on whether or not healing takes place. In these cases the form of treatment may not matter as much as preparing the body to be receptive to healing.

My personal belief is that for many cancers, psychological factors are of considerable importance. Unfortunately, many people are frightened by psychotherapy and immediately assume that there are no aspects of their past that could negatively impact their healing. Since this material is, for the most part, unconscious and denied, it is difficult for a person to accurately judge this within herself or himself. Seeing if you fit any of the cancer profile characteristics discussed below is a good starting point. A "not me" attitude also misses the opportunity that counseling offers to enhance life and help deal with the stress of having cancer, even if there are no psychological barriers to health. The debilitating emotions that accompany issues like fear of pain, fear of losing functions, fear of dying and of the unknown rock every cancer patient and their loved ones to their core. Yes, you can go through this alone or with the support of friends, but nothing beats a skilled therapist who is professionally trained to understand your feelings and is focused on helping you individually.

For many, there is still a stigma attached to receiving therapy. Many people equate psychotherapy with "There's something mentally wrong with me" or "I'm weak and inadequate." The reality is that everyone has acquired beliefs and behaviors early in life that no longer serve us. This says nothing bad about us, only that we are human. Therapy can help resolve emotional stresses that deplete our energy and immune system. It can help us live better, and obtain more of what we want in life. And people who are really living, who are doing what they really want, often do better. Therapy is for people who want to live life fully, with or without cancer. If I wanted to maximize my odds for survival, I would seek out a competent psychotherapist experienced in these issues to share in my journey.

Committing to Live

This book is designed to help people who want to live. In order to use this information effectively, the cancer patient must first answer the question: "Do I really want to live?" Other ways of asking this question are, "Do I find my life satisfying?" or "Do I usually look forward to the next day?" The inner will to live needs to come first to activate participation in the healing process at all levels—physical, emotional, and spiritual.

Some people are tired and have lost the zest for living. Dr. Lawrence LeShan, a psychologist who has worked extensively with cancer patients, makes the distinction that it is not that they want to die but that "they no longer want to live very much." If the commitment to living is absent or weak, the chances of survival are greatly reduced. If on some level you have lost your enthusiasm for life, then you may not have the energy to pursue all avenues for healing, and your immune system may be adversely affected. I believe this commitment to life is of paramount importance, yet it is often hard to tell if people have it or not. Cindy, for example, appeared to be happy and full of life, but there was a different story on the inside. On a deeper psychological level, Cindy's love for others was greater than for herself, and she had come to doubt she would achieve satisfaction in her life. Often, people with cancer are not consciously aware that a loss of hope has occurred. Cancer patients need to create an internal and external atmosphere conducive to healing. Because so much depends on commitment to life, it is an essential area of exploration for people with cancer.

Feelings

Emotions are one of the least understood and most important aspects of our well-being. Feelings are powerful electrochemical events in the body. When we are in touch with our feelings, and we allow them to come and go as they naturally occur, we are vibrant with the energy that they provide us. We learn through experiencing our emotions, and we are healthier because we are not creating blockages in our body's systems.

Feelings are meant to prepare the body for a certain activity. Fear, for example, releases adrenaline to prepare the body to fight or flee in order to defend itself. Feelings are natural processes that, when allowed to run their course, leave no residue of the experience other than a mental memory. This is not the case with feelings we do not want to experience. We often repress the experience of strong, uncomfortable feelings. We cut off the experience of unpleasant emotions through not breathing fully and by tightening our muscles in areas where the emotion would normally be felt.

These techniques cause the electrochemical feeling processes to stall, and the repressed emotional energies are stored in the muscle tissue of the body. There they continue to radiate their message on a subconscious level and can drain our energy and undermine the immune system. As previously stated, in Eastern medicine, these tightened areas of the body are seen as interrupting the flow of energy in the body, and they are where "dis-ease" originates.

For example, physically or psychologically abused children are not capable of handling the fear and terror of abuse. As a self-protective mechanism, the fear is repressed. Chronic fear has chemical components that diminish immune response, and years later these stored, unfelt feelings can still have immune-depleting effects.

But to say this does not mean we should start blaming ourselves. People should not be angry or impatient with themselves for having repressed emotions. We all avoid feelings for good reasons. These are natural self-preservation techniques that we employ until we are ready and capable of learning to handle our feelings in a new way.

Books

Neil Fiore, Ph.D., *The Road Back to Health: Coping with the Emotional Aspects of Cancer,* rev. ed. (Berkeley, CA: Celestial Arts, 1990).

Stuart Zelman, M.D., and David Bognar, *Human Operators Manual: How Feelings Work, a Psychological Primer* (Hartford, CT: n.p., 1991). Quickly and clearly explains how avoided emotions create pain and the potential for disease, then presents the process and rewards of releasing emotions. Available from authors for $10.95 at P.O. Box 8241, Manchester, CT 06040, 888-307-4482, or on their website: www.cancersurvival.com.

The Cancer Personality

Researchers have looked for personality characteristics shared by all cancer patients. Although no personality profile fits all people with cancer, some psychological traits and stressful events are common among many people who contract cancer. These include:

- having experienced a significant loss

- being overly critical toward oneself

- having a disturbed or emotionally sterile relationship with parents

- suppressing anger or strong emotions

- a loss of hope, depression, and being a self-sacrificing kind of person

Although no one personality factor is present for all people with cancer, for some types of cancers and for people with cancer in some age groups, psychological elements may be more of a factor.

Books

Lawrence LeShan, Ph.D., *You Can Fight for Your Life: Emotional Factors in the Causation of Cancer* (New York: M. Evans, 1980).

Lydia Temoshok, Ph.D., and Henry Dreher, *The Type C Connection: The Behavioral Links to Cancer and Your Health* (New York: Random House, 1992).

Cancer and Guilt

One pitfall of self-help psychology is the trap of blaming yourself for causing your illness. At any suggestion that an individual's psychology or beliefs may play a role in health, especially cancer, many people hear this as "I caused my disease." Dr. Bernie Siegel says that one reason people fall into the trap of blaming themselves for their cancer is preexisting guilt. Guilt is a pervasive emotion, although people are often not aware of it. Cindy told me that when she was a child, she often fantasized about being deathly ill with cancer and how her parents would be there for her, loving her and caring for her in the way all children want to be loved and cared for. Like most children who felt unloved, she thought she must have done some wrong, shamed herself, and then felt guilty. On some level it seemed Cindy's need to be loved, and her guilt, were being acted out within the drama of cancer.

The fact is, these are subtle and complex areas of thoughts, feelings, and a mixture of causes and effects that are best handled in therapy or small groups where any misinterpretation can be corrected by a professional counselor or psychotherapist.

A person's psychological makeup, developed during childhood, can weaken the immune system. If, psychologically, he lacks a zest for living, this could be a factor in having cancer, but it does not mean that the individual is to blame. We usually associate cause with conscious choice. To be at fault is to cause something willfully. But, as Dr. LeShan says, no one consciously chooses to have cancer. On the other hand, if a person smokes cigarettes, knowing it can cause lung cancer, and it does, did that person cause her lung cancer? Quite possibly, yes. If a person unknowingly is exposed to large doses of a carcinogen, has that person caused his or her own cancer? No, most people would assume the exposure was to blame, not the person. If the person, through the normal activity of living, develops unconscious beliefs and emotional states that stress the immune system and then becomes ill, is the person to blame? No, she did not choose to have these beliefs; they developed as a natural response to living.

Holistic medicine maintains that there can be many contributing factors or causes for any disease, including cancer. As the Chinese book of wisdom, the *I Ching*, encourages people to remember in situations like this, "No blame."

Learning to Love Self

One of the personality traits associated with cancer patients is lack of self-appreciation, or being critical of oneself. But self-love is a spiritual topic for cancer patents, because love is one of the most common and central attributes ascribed to God and potentially one of the most important qualities necessary for people to heal.

Self-esteem is acknowledging our worth. When we love ourselves, we are gentle, patient, and understanding with ourselves. We like who we are and we treat ourselves well. We allow ourselves the time and space to grow, to enjoy life and have pleasure. We operate in a loving, calm state, and the world is loving around us.

Why is it, then, that most people do not feel self-loving but instead career like pinballs from one event to another, grasping for something or someone in order to feel okay about themselves? The truth is that a variety of mental barriers prevent us from loving ourselves: limiting messages from parents and families; social pressures and codes; religious teachings that devalue the self.

Barriers to self-love usually begin with parental training. Children who are not taught that they are good and okay become dependent on others for their sense of self-worth and self-acceptance. The culture we live in also has all sorts of prerequisites to self-worth. We are okay if we have certain things, look a certain way, or exhibit certain attributes or characteristics. To make matters worse, some religions have taught that loving oneself is a sin, a sign of selfishness, an impertinence before God. The truth is that we are naturally, at our core, always good and worth loving. It is a basic attribute of people: that love exists at the core of our being.

Fortunately, mistaken beliefs can be replaced with more freeing beliefs that allow people to like and love themselves more fully (see "Affirmations," in chapter 6).

Isn't a belief in your self-worth better, more productive, and more satisfying than a belief that discounts your worthiness? Self-doubt and criticism create stress that can negatively affect the immune system. Conversely, learning self-acceptance and self-love may help immunity and, at the very least, provide a more enjoyable life experience.

Books

Bernie S. Siegel, M.D., *Love, Medicine, & Miracles: Lessons Learned About Self-Healing from a Surgeon's Experience with Exceptional Patients* (New York: Harper & Row, 1986) and *Peace, Love, & Healing: Bodymind Communication and the Path to Self-Healing: An Exploration* (New York: Harper & Row, 1989).

Stuart Zelman, M.D., and David Bognar, *Human Operators Manual: How Feelings Work, a Psychological Primer* (Hartford, CT: n.p., 1991). Contains an exercise for building self-esteem, also sound information on learning to love oneself. Available from the authors for $10.95 at P.O. Box 8241, Manchester, CT 06040, 888-307-4482, www.cancersurvival.com.

Finding a Therapist

Though there are many remarkable and effective psychotherapies, they are often represented by mediocre therapists. It is important to find a therapist who is skilled at guiding and supporting you through the process of change. Finding a good therapist is like finding a good car mechanic—and they are about as common.

Knowing the basic differences among psychiatrists, psychologists, and other psychotherapists is a good place to start. *Psychotherapist* or *therapist* is a general term used to describe any person, regardless of training, who is in the business of providing psychological therapy.

Psychiatrists are psychotherapists who have completed standard medical doctors' training and an internship at a psychiatric hospital. The amount of psychological training a psychiatrist receives depends on courses available during medical school and on what the doctor chooses to learn on her or his own after being granted a medical degree. Psychiatrists, being trained in medicine, are the only therapists who can prescribe medications in the treatment of emotional problems.

Psychologists are people who have completed four years of graduate training in psychology (attaining a Ph.D.). Master's-level psychologists are those who have completed two years of graduate level work in psychology, although some programs require only one year.

Social workers have attained a master's degree in social work; some social work schools offer little or no clinical training, while others have well-developed courses in counseling and therapeutic intervention. Social workers can be certified and/or licensed. In the past, social workers were trained largely to provide social services in agencies. Increasingly, social workers seek additional psychotherapeutic training and establish private practices.

Psychologists and psychiatrists can receive third-party insurance payments. Social workers can receive third-party payments, but depending on the insurance policy, their services may or may not be covered. Therapy provided by master's-level or nondegreed therapists can sometimes be billed through a supervising Ph.D. Check with your insurance carrier for your policy's specifics.

Lay therapists and *nondegreed therapists* are people who have a desire or natural talent to do psychotherapy. They may have some general training in psychology or training in a particular type of therapy, but they do not have professional accreditation. Nondegreed therapists can be as helpful as degreed therapists, except in cases of severe disorders and people requiring medication. There appear to be as many incompetent therapists with degrees as there are without them, which makes it all the more difficult to locate a therapist right for you.

How much do therapists cost? Generally, nondegreed therapists charge anywhere from $40 to $60 per hour, master's-level social workers a little more, psychologists $70 to $100 per hour, and psychiatrists $100 and up. Fees will vary from person to person and state to state, and may be higher than listed here. Insurance may pay nothing, 50 percent, and occasionally 80 percent. If you are in an HMO, therapy may be less expensive. Your challenge may be to convince the HMO that you need an outside therapist, because your chances of finding a competent therapist trained in dealing with cancer patients within an HMO are slim.

Weekly therapy may appear to be a costly item until you consider the pain and suffering that can be alleviated and the satisfaction it can help you obtain in life. Therapy can be absolutely cost-effective, if you find a good therapist.

You may have to shop around. As Lawrence LeShan says, you want the grown-ups, the experienced older therapists (see interview, below). Do not be embarrassed to ask questions, or feel intimidated; you are choosing someone with whom you will have an intimate personal relationship. When calling to inquire, explain that you are looking for a therapist and that you want to find one who is right for you. Explain why you want to see a therapist, and ask if they have had experience assisting people with life-threatening diseases. You can ask whatever questions you want. Ask what questions they would ask if they were looking for a therapist for the same purpose. Then ask them the same questions. If they sound put off by your questions, you are probably better off with some one else. Don't forget to ask about cost and insurance arrangements.

Use your intuition. If a person sounds good to you, make an

appointment. Have an initial consultation with more than one thera-pist. Initial consultations sometimes are free, or discounted. You may spend a little extra money, but finding a good therapist can result in greater progress and satisfaction, using less time and money in the long run. When you meet the therapist for the first time, trust your instincts. Does the therapist listen well? Can you relate to this per-son? Do you trust him? Do you sense that she understands you, your goals, and what you are saying?

After you have picked a therapist, work with him for a couple of months. Do you sense a change? Do you think that you are making progress? Do you feel good about what is happening? The tricky part is that sometimes progress includes pain, and we often blame the therapist for what we experience. It is sometimes hard to tell when we are running from bad therapy or from the result of good therapy. Good therapy, however, is usually marked by slow and supportive res-olution of emotional issues paced to the individual. Good therapy is usually productive, even though it may be scary. Good therapy feels right. Trusting your instincts and results are your best bet.

Book

Lawrence LeShan, Ph.D., *Cancer as a Turning Point: A Handbook for People with Cancer, Their Families, and Health Professionals* (New York: Dutton/ Penguin, 1989). Contains LeShan's suggestions for finding a therapist; also see his suggestions in the interview below.

Bioenergetics

Bioenergetics is one of six Reichian therapies. Wilhelm Reich was a psychiatrist, a student of Freud, and a scientist who came to believe in the existence of a potent natural energy that he called the "X-force" or "orgone energy." His pioneering work made him the father of today's body energy therapies. At least six therapies have grown out of his work, including bioenergetics.

Bioenergetics was developed by psychiatrists Alexander Lowen and John Pierrakos. It is based on the understanding that feelings are electrochemical events in the body and that tensing muscles is one of the primary techniques people use to avoid experiencing their feelings.

These "stored" energies remain in the body but can be released during psychotherapy with the aid of emotion-specific body postures. In theory, this can aid in healing by relieving emotional and psychological blocks, which in turn reduce the continual stress on the immune system.

Book

Alexander Lowen, M.D., *Bioenergetics* (New York: Penguin, 1975).

Organization

International Institute for Bioenergetic Analysis
144 E. 36th Street, Suite 1A
New York, NY 10016
Phone: 212-532-7742
Website: www.bioenergetic-therapy.com

LeShan Approach

Lawrence LeShan, Ph.D., is one of the grand masters of psychology, and the pioneer of psychological intervention for cancer. He is a psychologist who first began working with terminal cancer patients using classic Freudian therapy techniques, only to find, as he openly states, "They all died." LeShan learned that the traditional psychotherapy approach (searching for pathology and its roots) was ineffective.

In researching the problem further, he noticed that a majority of his clients had lost their enthusiasm for life. They had reached a point where they no longer believed they would be able to achieve the kind of satisfying life they desired. LeShan developed a new approach. It entailed helping people search for what would be a zestful and enthusiastic life for them—helping them to, as he puts it, "find their song."

With this form of therapy, a majority of his terminal clients went into remission, or their cancer otherwise resolved. Remarkable, but not unscientific, according to LeShan. To him, and to those who practice his form of therapy, it is simply a matter of relieving stress on the immune system and allowing it to improve its ability to function.

LeShan emphatically states that it is not a matter of people creating their own reality (see "Creating Your Reality?" in chapter 8). He is critical of unskilled therapists who leave their clients feeling guilty that they were in some way responsible for their cancer.

Practitioner

Lawrence LeShan, Ph.D.
263 West End Avenue
New York, NY 10023
Phone: 212-724-5802

Book

Lawrence LeShan, Ph.D., *Cancer as a Turning Point: A Handbook for People with Cancer, Their Families, and Health Professionals* (New York: Dutton/Penguin, 1989). An absolute must-read for people with cancer.

Psychosynthesis

Psychosynthesis, developed by Italian psychiatrist Roberto Assagioli, is the type of therapy used by Alice Hopper-Epstein to heal herself of cancer, as described in her book *Mind, Fantasy, and Healing: One Woman's Journey from Conflict and Illness to Wholeness and Health* (New York: Delacorte Press, 1989).

According to psychosynthesis, we all originate from a positively oriented spiritual core, and all aspects of the self, having originated from that core, must also have a positive intent. Those aspects of self that seem to be negative are understood as operating on learned beliefs that were formed to help protect us in some way, and hence they have a positive intent.

The therapy consists, among other things, of the therapist guiding the client in a light trance journey through the inner self, accompanied by a source of inner wisdom. Having experienced this therapy, I can attest to its effectiveness and to how remarkable and productive this inner journey can be.

Book

Alice Hopper-Epstein, Ph.D., *Mind, Fantasy, and Healing: One Woman's Journey from Conflict and Illness to Wholeness and Health* (New York: Delacorte Press, 1989).

Organization

Association for the Advancement of Psychosynthesis
P.O. Box 597
Amherst, MA 01004-0597
Phone: 413-253-6971

Rebirthing

Rebirthing, like many feeling-release therapies, relies on slow and steady breathing to reestablish a natural connection to feelings that are being avoided through incomplete breathing. Slow, complete breathing reconnects a person to repressed feelings and then allows the person to release them by simply experiencing them. Rebirthing is commonly misunderstood to be solely concerned with those feelings that may have resulted from birth trauma. Although rebirthing can be used for this, it also can be used to release the full range of unexpressed trauma built up throughout a person's life. Rebirthing is a quick, direct therapy for those who want to release stored emotions.

Book

Leonard Orr and Sondra Ray, *Rebirthing in the New Age* (Berkeley, CA: Celestial Arts, 1983).

Website

Breathe: The International Breathwork Journal homepage
www.users.znet.co.uk/rmoore

Simonton Approach

O. Carl Simonton, M.D., is a radiation oncologist who is another pioneer in the psychological treatment of cancer. Simonton pioneered the use of imagery and uses techniques for gaining access to inner wisdom, the knowledgeable aspect of self useful for providing healing information (see "Internal Wisdom," chapter 8). Dr. Simonton is the author of books and tapes well worth inspection, and he currently operates the Simonton Cancer Center. The center offers a five-and-a-half-day program of psychological intervention and support for cancer patients. Although the program is somewhat costly, some insurances will cover it in part. Clients can be confident they are participating in a state-of-the-art program.

Books

O. Carl Simonton, M.D., and Reid Henson, with Brenda Hampton, *The Healing Journey: The Simonton Center Program for Achieving Physical, Mental, and Spiritual Health* (New York: Bantam Books, 1992).

O. Carl Simonton, M.D., Stephanie Matthews-Simonton, and James L. Creighton, *Getting Well Again: A Step-by-Step, Self-Help Guide to Overcoming Cancer for Patients and Their Families* (Los Angeles, CA: J. P. Tarcher, 1978).

Organization

Simonton Cancer Center
P.O. Box 890
Pacific Palisades, CA 90272
Phone: 800-338-2360 (for publications and tapes)
Phone: 800-459-3424 (for information on five-day intensive workshop)

Videotape

The Healing Process. A videotape interview of Dr. Simonton, available from Thinking Allowed for $49.95. Phone 800-999-4415.

Chapter Resources

Books

Joan Borysenko, Ph.D., *Minding the Body, Mending the Mind* (New York: Bantam Books, 1987).

Joan Borysenko, Ph.D., and Miroslav Borysenko, *The Power of the Mind to Heal* (Carson, CA: Hay House, 1994).

Norman Cousins, *Anatomy of an Illness as Perceived by the Patient* (New York: Bantam, 1981).

Norman Cousins, *Head First: The Biology of Hope and the Healing Power of the Human Spirit* (New York: Penguin, 1990).

Lawrence LeShan, Ph.D., *Cancer as a Turning Point: A Handbook for People with Cancer, Their Families, and Health Professionals* (New York: Dutton/ Penguin, 1989). Contains a chapter entitled "Meditation for Change and Growth."

Steven E. Locke, M.D., and Douglas Colligan, *The Healer Within: The New Medicine of Mind and Body* (New York: New American Library, 1986).

Kenneth R. Pelletier, *Mind as Healer, Mind as Slayer: A Holistic Approach to Preventing Stress Disorders* (New York: Delacorte Press, 1977).

Jimmie C. Holland and Julia H. Rowland, eds., *Handbook of Psychooncology* (New York: Oxford University Press, 1989).

Organization

Simonton Cancer Center
P.O. Box 890
Pacific Palisades, CA 90272
Phone: 800-338-2360

Offers a catalog of books and tapes on mind-body therapy for cancer patients.

Interview with
Lawrence LeShan, Ph.D.

on the Psychology of Cancer, Stress and the Immune System, Enthusiasm to Live, Finding a Therapist, and Fulfilling Your Dreams

Lawrence LeShan, Ph.D., is a pioneering psychologist who worked extensively with cancer patients for over forty years. He believes that many people suffering from cancer have lost their hope of ever achieving a satisfying life. He believes that combining the power of "finding their song" with other healing methods may mean the difference between life and death. He is a prolific author whose works include: *Cancer as a Turning Point: A Handbook for People with Cancer, Their Families, and Health Professionals*; *You Can Fight for Your Life: Emotional Factors in the Causation of Cancer*; *The Mechanic and the Gardener: How to Use the Holistic Revolution in Medicine*; *How to Meditate: A Guide to Self-Discovery*; *The Medium, The Mystic, and the Physicist: Toward a General Theory of the Paranormal*; *Alternate Realities: The Search for the Full Human Being*; *The Science of the Paranormal: The Next Frontier*; *Einstein's Space and Van Gogh's Sky: Physical Reality and Beyond* (with Henry Margenau). Although I had heard about Dr. Lawrence LeShan, I didn't discover his book *Cancer as a Turning Point* soon enough for Cindy to read. He has the wisdom, skill, and presence of the quintessential therapist, and he is beyond doubt one of that special breed of wise old masters of psychology.

How did you determine that in the 1800s, the relationship between cancer and psychological factors had been commonly accepted?

One of the most interesting things about this field is that up until the 1900s the idea that psychological factors played a part in cancer was simply accepted by everybody. I went through the major cancer textbooks—*major* meaning those that had gone to three editions—in English. Of thirty-seven of them, thirty-six said that of course emotional life factors played a part. In that [era] it was useless information; they had no tools to intervene further, with psychiatry having been developed to a descriptive phase, and so the knowledge was lost. It just dropped out of the literature.

The major textbook of the middle of the nineteenth century was a book by Walter Walsh, who was the great authority of that time, entitled *The Nature and Treatment of Cancer.* It said that if you had a family with a high cancer incidence, you should take special precautions. For example, you should not take a job with high stress, such as medicine, law, or business. You should have a job with little stress, such as the army, navy, or the church. This was the advice he gave, but if you think about what it means, it is a curiously modern viewpoint. If you have a genetic factor and a long-term psychological stress, these two tend to eventuate in a much higher level of cancer.

The field dropped out of existence for about fifty years, from 1900 to 1950. Although there was one major study—a woman named Lida Evans analyzed one hundred women with breast cancer. Outside of that it disappeared.

Then in 1950 a new group started to come in all over America. They were clinical psychologists and psychiatrists with brand new tools. What they found was very similar to what had been found in the early nineteenth century. There were no tests, but you had dedicated physicians who, having no tools, no CAT scans, no X rays, had to listen to their patients. What they heard was that cancer tended to occur in a context, in a context of the loss of hope of ever achieving a real meaningful, zestful life—a life of enthusiasm. They found this over and over, starting with the first reports in 1799. Not always. Nobody ever claimed, except the real kooks, that emotional factors *caused* cancer—that was ridiculous. Emotional factors don't cause it, and they don't cure it. Nobody should ever get the silly idea that they are either responsible for the cancer or responsible for getting better. It's nonsense.

But psychological factors play a *part.* The psychological factors affect the body chemistry. The cells swim in the body chemistry, it is their environment, and they do affect the appearance and prognosis of cancer. There may be only a small effect. We don't know how large it is, but suppose it's only 5 percent. Think what a difference 5 percent can make in a hard-fought election. This is very similar to what we have here with modern medicine and cancer. They are simply hard-fought elections, and often, even if it's only a small part, [these factors] can play a decisive role.

Could you say a little bit more about the emotional life and history of the average cancer patient?

What we know today about the psychological factors is that in a considerable proportion of cancers patients, there has been a loss of hope, loss of belief that they will ever have the kind of life that makes you want to get out of bed in the morning. Sometimes this occurs after the death of a spouse. The death of a spouse, whether male or female, tends to really increase the likelihood of getting cancer. Another way you see it very clearly is in forced retirement. No matter what age you retire people, the next few years show a tremendous surge in cancer. For example, going through life, the cancer rate increases very gradually. Suppose at seventy years old you have an automatic retirement age, then the cancer mortality rate shows a big leap for five years, but suppose people automatically retire at sixty-five, then the big leap comes here.

We even [saw this in a group that] retired at *thirty-five.* Right after World War II, there was a theory that people who had been enthusiastic members of the Nazi party were not very nice people and shouldn't be allowed to work in the German bureaucratic system. They were told they could never work in it again. A German sociologist named Joyce Fall followed what happened. The same tremendously high peak of the cancer mortality rate.

You can show it in a dozen different ways, for example, by marital status. The marital status where this has happened most often is the death of a spouse. That is the highest cancer mortality rate, at any age. The next is divorce. The next is married [people who] made the relationship but [then felt they] lost it. The next is single where they haven't made the relationship. This is exactly what the cancer mortality rate follows, and it's what you would expect—at the loss of a major relationship, loss of hope.

We have gathered together dozens of statistics of this kind, and we found they all lead to the same point: that when you have a group where life events indicate to them that they will never again enjoy meaningful enthusiasm, joy, and zest, the cancer defense mechanism tends to operate less strongly, leaving them more vulnerable.

The viewpoint we are working on today is pretty much as follows: that everybody gets cancer dozens of times a day; we have billions of cells that multiply, divide, slip over the line; they lose their coherence with themselves and with the rest of the body and become cancer cells. But the body has a mechanism, and nobody has the faintest idea what it is. We call it the "cancer defense mechanism" because it is chic, and you feel "in" if you use the correct words. We say it is part of the immune system—whatever that means. It doesn't mean much, but it makes us feel like we know something.

For example, if you try to give cancer to people where the cancer defense mechanism is intact, you can't do it. It is hard to get volunteers for these experiments, but we did. A number of people in prison with very long sentences were asked if they would volunteer to be in a very dangerous experiment, and if they survived they would get parole. We injected them with the most virulent combinations of cancer cells we could find, but nobody got cancer. Only local infection and local irritation that when left alone went away in three days.

As long as the cancer defense mechanism is intact, it takes care of these cells that lose their coherence. When it breaks down the cells develop into cancer. The strength of this mechanism is set by some very complicated genetic pattern. Again, we have no particular idea about this [pattern] except that it is a real one. It can be weakened by various things, such as coal tar products, which is why we advise people to stop smoking. Or by environmental pollutants, which is why we hope to hell the government will start doing something about it. Solar radiation and the breakdown of the ozone layer is going to produce a lot more of it. It can also be very much weakened by the loss of hope. When you lose that, the immune system stops fighting so hard, cancer cells slip through that barrier, and you have a much greater tendency to develop cancer.

This, of course, raises the question, What would happen if they regained the hope? Would the cancer defense mechanism be strengthened again? There was no way to know this in advance. You could try psychotherapy, but it had had no success in helping people with cancer. It is not surprising, since it wasn't built for that.

Psychotherapy was built for something else entirely, for problems of personality, memory, perception, and feelings. Every experienced therapist [has] had patients that, after a long successful therapy, developed cancer. So we began to devise a therapy approach that was different from the standard one and was specifically designed for cancer patients. We said, "Okay, there was a loss of hope about ever achieving a meaningful life." And where does this hope come from? This hope really comes when you have a chance of saying, "I as an individual will sing my own special song in life, beat out my own music, do what I am built for as a person." We began to design a therapy built on that to help the person seek their own special song. The questions we worked with were no longer the usual three questions of psychotherapy: (1) What's wrong with you? (2) How did you get that way? What is the hidden cause—the oedipal conflict or loss of contact with your inner child or whatever the shtick is at the moment? (3) What can we do about it? Slowly we began to devise a new kind of therapy built on two different questions: What is right with you as an individual? And what can we do about it?

We found that the older models of therapy hadn't worked for cancer. In our experience we found some very special factors in the cancer patient. These weren't neurotic people or sick people as a general rule; there was no common personality profile, nothing general about them except that a very large percentage, 70 to 80 percent, had really lost hope of achieving an enjoyable life. Life was just an endless getting up in the morning and going on with what you were doing. No reward beyond that. So we began to design a therapy to help each person seek for what was *right* for them, to create life that would make them want to get up in the morning.

If there is one word that sums up our knowledge about stimulating the immune system, it is *enthusiasm*. It is nothing that can be faked. Many people had to really embark *full-heartedly* on this search for the kind of activities, relationships, and creativity that really turned them on. It is almost as if the immune system looks up and says, "Here is an individual worth fighting for." And frequently, though not always, the immune system begins to operate at a higher level. We see this result by the [tendency of these people] to have a much better [response] to medical treatment and medical programs that they hadn't been responding to [before]. This is something to be done not *instead* of a medical treatment, but to *augment* medical treatment.

When I first started out, and for the first fifteen years or so, I worked only with people who were absolutely medically hopeless. People who, from any medical viewpoint, had been told, "Don't buy any magazine subscriptions, and make your will." One hundred percent of my patients died using the older methods of therapy. Using this [different] method of therapy with the same population, about 50 percent began to respond to the medical treatment in new ways. We tell people that we make no promises, but [this therapy] will do two things. One, it will change the color of your life. You'll want to fight for your life. And, it will tend to augment your immune system and will help the medical treatment.

There is a real difference in tone between the two types of therapy. I have been a patient in both types of therapy and a therapist in both types of therapy. There is a very real difference between spending two years trying to find out all the things that are wrong with you and two years trying to find out all the things that are right with you. It is really much more of an adventure opening up, a looking at the best of one's self. How one functions most fully and joyously. Sometimes you have to go into the past very deeply but always in the context of how the past is blocking your future, how the past is blocking your real enjoyment.

What are most important questions for cancer patients to ask themselves?

What part of myself is undernourished? What part of myself—physical, emotional, spiritual—have I given the least to? What dreams have I left unfulfilled behind me? What would I regret most not having done? What kinds of activities have given [me] those wonderful moments where I suddenly look up and three hours have gone by—I have missed lunch, but I'm charged up? When do I have a *good* tired feeling, not a *blah* tired feeling? And what has kept me from doing them? Frequently people feel, "Well, I certainly can't do it, I can't earn my living at it"; and second, "I am probably a pretty unpleasant person at heart and I wouldn't like it very much if I found my own dreams"; and third, "It's so complicated." One said, "Doctor, you don't know. I am a very complex guy. I need things I can't have together—it is sort of like I want to be a hermit with a harem—it's too complicated." I work with literally thousands of patients with this approach, [and in thirty-five years] I have never had anybody with a dream that couldn't be fulfilled.

A typical example where it looked like it couldn't be fulfilled—there was this man in his sixties who came to see me, named Mack. He knew what he wanted, he wanted to be a physician. Obviously an impossible dream. [I worked with him to find out what "being a physician" meant to him. It meant that] people would come with their problems, and he would have the resources and training to solve their problems.

How did Mack fulfill his dream? While driving to Florida from New York, Mack passed a lot of exits to the resort cities, and he got off at one that said "Tourist Information." [He got a job solving people's vacation problems.] I drove down there once to see him. A family came in asking him to make hotel reservations for them. In five minutes, doing the best psychiatric interview I have ever seen, Mack helped them figure out what they wanted out of the vacation. They had never talked about these things, but he drew it out of them. He then made three phone calls and sent them on their way.

I have never seen a more fulfilled man. He's living out his dream fully, richly, completely. The only problem he has is with his boss, who keeps telling him this is a nine-to-five job; you don't have to show up at seven and leave at eight. It is this kind of thing that I see over and over again. When people begin to understand what kind of relating and creating would really turn them on, it is always available, and it can always be done.

Do you believe that cancer patients have [unconsciously] lost the will to live? That their cancer is part of determining whether they will live or die?

I have never known anybody who, at any level, wanted to have cancer. I have known people that didn't want to live very much anymore, whose will to live had been weakened. But I have never known anybody who chose cancer. None of my patients really wanted to die; they really didn't want to live, but they really didn't want to die. There is a fundamental difference there.

I don't think people choose their cancer. I think that is one of the most difficult aspects of this whole field. Some amateurs have said the patient causes their cancer and they are responsible for it. Unfortunately, some of the major textbooks in this field and the most widely read books are written by amateurs, people who are highly trained medical experts in other fields but not this one. They leave the patients feeling guilty. I have never had a patient who wound up feeling guilty.

In the first few years of our lives we have to come to some very major decisions: What kind of a person am I? What is a good person? How do I relate to other people? How do other people relate to me? What kind of a world is it? We come to these with limited experience, with an unfinished brain, and we are kind of stuck with these decisions. Later, events happen: the death of a spouse, retirement, loss of a job. Sometimes events so interact with our early understanding of the world that we lose hope. Not a depression, but a loss of hope. At that point our defense mechanisms stop fighting so hard, and it is hard to stay alive.

We live on a madly spinning planet. It tends to spin us off into the outer darkness. We have to hold onto it with meaning, with work, with relationships.

How do people find a therapist with this new viewpoint? Some people might go out and get a lot of these self-help books, figuring they'll figure out on their own why they've lost their will to live. Could you say something about that?

There are some people who can work on it on their own, but they are fairly few. It doesn't mean they are more intelligent, more creative, or stronger; it just means that the combination of circumstances makes it possible. Most of us need help to do this, to turn our lives around, to make the cancer a turning point in our life.

I advise people to shop around among the therapists in their area. First, get the grown-ups, the seasoned ones who have been around awhile. Second, you should like them. There should be a good chemistry; otherwise it is much harder. Third, say "I want to work from the viewpoint of what is right with me and not what is wrong with me." Sometimes [my readers] give their therapist a paperback copy of the book *Cancer as a Turning Point* and ask, "Can you work from this viewpoint? Will you make a contract with me to work on what's right with me? And when you forget, I will remind you, and when I forget, you remind me."

After you find a therapist who fits that and who is mature enough to say, "Yes, let's try that," then you have got a good chance. And I have had some very good feedback results from parts of Europe and this country, people using that kind of approach.

One patient said to me, "I know what you're doing. All my life I have worn pretty good clothes. I go to Brooks Brothers and wear good suits. But once I went to a really good tailor and had him design a suit of clothes for me from the ground up." And he said, "Boy, those were fighting clothes—I felt good in those. That's what you're talking about with therapy." He was absolutely right.

In Cancer as a Turning Point *you said you learned that those patients using a wider approach to dealing with the disease—from the physical, emotional, and spiritual—did better. What did you mean by that?*

I dealt with the psychological, while they were getting medical treatment. I never would work with anyone not under medical care. And of the things we found out is that—I learned this largely from my patients—the best seem to be those that went beyond me. For example, I began looking at their nutrition and exercise to find a nutrition program that was right for *them*. There is a diet that is very popular in the cancer field known as the "macrobiotic diet." I have known people that did beautifully on it, and I have known people who have died on it. It is right for some and wrong for others—just as is any style of living, way of relating, way of creating. What type of diet is right for you? What kind of food makes you feel good and energetic and [is food] that you don't crash on afterward? What kind of food is addictive and therefore you must stay away from it? And the same thing for an exercise program. Just because jogging is popular it doesn't mean you take up jogging. You experiment until you find the way that feels most right for you.

Also, there is the spiritual. This is, of course, the hardest word in the English language to define. One way [to define it] is those disciplines of prayer and meditation that make you feel at home in the world. You have these wonderful moments of knowing that you are part of the cosmos and cannot be separated from it. Your loneliness and alienation are simply illusion. Whether you call this "Christ consciousness" or "cosmic consciousness" or "satori" or any one of a thousand things, it doesn't much matter—they take long hard work and discipline.

There is another aspect to the spiritual that is particularly important for us as Westerners. In the Western spiritual tradition we have always been much more concerned with what you *did* than how you *felt*. St. John of the Cross put it [this way]: "If you are in ecstasy as deep as that of St. Paul and a sick man needed a cup of soup, it would be better for you to return from that ecstasy and bring him the soup for love's sake." In the Western spiritual tradition, doing for others has to come after doing for yourself. No patient who has finished with me isn't doing something like this—I have got patients working as volunteers one night a week with the Big Brothers or Big Sisters, peace organizations. You find that more than one person says, "It [doing for others] feeds a part of me that I never knew was hungry." This is what I mean by the spiritual today. The fullest, richest life will be taken care of not only by the physical and psychological, but also the spiritual.

There are no guarantees in this. All there is in this approach is a chance to fight for the best and the fullest of yourself and to get the most out of your life before you die. It also strengthens your immune system, but that isn't the goal. The goal isn't to increase the number of fluttering of leaves on a calendar, but to increase the richness, the extension of life. There is an old medieval manuscript, the Zohar, that says, "God's purpose is not to add years to your life but life to your years." This is what we are talking about here.

When you say it is a good idea for people to work on the spiritual, most people think of a church. What avenue do you suggest to people to explore the spiritual?

As they explore themselves, I help people explore the spiritual. Not in terms of what they are supposed to do, and certainly not in terms of church activities, although that is right for many people. I explore in terms of: What are their hidden springs of will and wish and desire? What do they need to turn them on more fully? What do they need to make them feel they are flowering as fully as a rose in the spring? One of the things they find, very often with great surprise, is that part of it is their social being; they are a social human being. It is more than yourself and your family. We are a part of our community or world or our planet. When this comes up, I then encourage people, just as with exercise, to experiment until they find the right style for them, and this changes from time to time, too. With diet, with ways of being creative, and with ways of expressing the spiritual part [I advise people] to experiment with various ideas.

There is so much need in our society. We need desperately to save the ozone layer and the whales, feed the homeless, and God knows what. There are tremendous needs. Every human being is needed. What is the best way for you to put your ounces of weight against the tremendous need so that you feel most satisfied? There are people that feel very unsatisfied working for whales and for the homeless. For everyone there is some need that fits them like two pieces of a jigsaw puzzle.

How does one know if they are in the "getting well mode" or "the dying mode," and what do you mean by that?

What we have been talking about so far are people in the sick mode. When someone is in the sick mode, you do everything possible to help them get better. You urge them and work with them to get the best medical treatment, the best physical treatment, the best psychological treatment, the best of everything. Sometimes a person reaches a point of deep psychological exhaustion that almost feels like a physical adrenal exhaustion. It's not, but it feels like it. There is nothing left to fight with. At that point, the approach of the therapist and the person himself have to change. Not, how do I *change* things, but how do I *understand* things? What do I have to do to complete my life, to go peacefully and to give up the hatreds and sadness? We do this by understanding it.

One man came to me, and his mother was dying in the hospital. He said, "I go to the hospital, and we sit and try to talk, and she complains about the food, the nursing, the pain. I leave and feel unsatisfied, and she feels unsatisfied, and I don't know what to do." I gave him some advice. The mother is clearly in the dying mode. After she died he came back with the following story.

The next time he saw his mother, he said, "Tell me, Mom, what was it like growing up as a girl in a little Ohio town in 1915?" They began to talk, and he kept asking things like, "What was the most important decision you ever made, and why?" "What was the time you were most really you?" "What would you liked to have changed in your life?" They began to talk more and more, and as she was talking she would say things like, "Oh, that was the reason I did that," or, "I understand what that was about." Very shortly the complaints about the pain and food began to drop out, and they began to talk more and more about the serious things her life was really about. And he began to tell her things that he had never spoken of before. He began to tape-record some of these for her grandchildren. One night she took the tape recorder and recorded a message to be read at her funeral, telling him how much this had meant to her and how her whole dying process changed.

The task of dying time is to understand the meaning of our life, to see the total symphony, to put the parts together that rise and swell. When someone is dying, what you do is help them to understand the meaning of their life. What *they* have to do is to understand more completely, to forgive themselves for the things that have happened to them, and to forgive others so that they can go peacefully.

If you had one message for cancer patients, what would it be?

No matter how long your life is going to be, try to get the most out of it. When we seek for the best in ourselves, we are also seeking ultimately for the best in our relationships with other people—which does *not* make us into hermits or narcissists; it really makes us into someone who lives fully on all levels. And this enriches whatever period of life you've got left and also strengthens the cancer defense mechanism and the medical program you're in.

[All interviews have been edited for length and clarity.]

Dr. LeShan resides in Manhattan and can be reached at 212-724-5802 for consultations and refereral services.

Part 4

Spirituality and Mortality

8

Cancer and Spirituality

Many people report that cancer is an ironic gift, a disease that threatens their physical existence while calling on them to explore their true nature and the meaning of their lives. For many, this means exploring what is really important to them and finding or reconnecting to a Higher Power. For some, it becomes an avenue for healing, an opportunity for discovering a source of healing and peace within, and sometimes finding that this results in a remission or cure. It is important to note that the success rate for a physical cure using psychospiritual approaches is considered to be low. It is true, however, that patients who believe there is a spiritual force tend to live longer.

Dr. O. Carl Simonton, a radiation oncologist who pioneered the use of imagery and who advocates using our spiritual resources to assist in healing, observes,

> The role of spiritual beliefs in stress management has been, to me, virtually ignored, and it's huge. Our beliefs about our nature, our beliefs about the creative forces in the universe, our beliefs about the meaning of life, our beliefs about death—all have a huge impact on the way we live our lives. And we can explore our beliefs in these areas in the same way that we can explore our beliefs about anything else, and we can determine a relative health value. And especially for people dealing with serious illness, where death is a real probability, coming to terms with issues of death is very important for freeing up energy to live life.

Eastern spiritual thought teaches an idea found in many religions, including Christianity, that there is an all-loving God, divine light, or creative intelligence within us. If this divine spark or God essence is within us, then it is not something we have to achieve or to become, because it is something we already have. It is simply a matter of removing the barrier to gaining access to that force within.

Dr. Bernie Siegel says that it is a natural force within us that does the healing. If we didn't have the natural ability to heal, surgeons would cut us open, and our incisions wouldn't heal. Advocates of spiritual healing believe that our bodies are intimately interwoven with this vast, relatively untapped, higher intelligence some call God, which does the healing.

While physical healing refers to the cure of a physical ailment, another concept of healing encompasses the healing of a person on a psycho-spiritual level. Here, healing takes on a new meaning, the healing of the soul. From this perspective, the healing journey means finding or rediscovering the spiritual core or higher power within. This includes the healing or resolution of past, unresolved emotional issues and, on a spiritual level, finding the peace within where there is no longer unease or fear, just the loving connection with the true self.

Books

Richard Carlson, Ph.D., and Benjamin Shield, eds., *Healers on Healing* (Los Angeles, CA: J. P. Tarcher, 1989). Excellent collection of thirty-seven essays, by some of the world's most well-known experts on healing.

Creating Your Reality?

There has been much controversy and confusion over the idea that people may in some way be responsible for creating their cancer (see "Cancer and Guilt," chapter 7). Some of this confusion seems due to an increased awareness of the new age concept of "manifesting your reality." To try and understand this issue, it is important to know how it has developed.

In recent years, one popular area of spiritual exploration has been the concept that our consciousness and thoughts interact with the unified field of energy some call God and that this creates, over time, what takes place on the physical level. There is, in fact, support for this theory in quantum physics.

Confusion arises when people interpret this process to mean "I am solely responsible for the creation of my reality." This appears unlikely, if you entertain the concept of what Dr. Carl Jung called the "collective unconscious." Imagine that people's minds are "nonlocal"— not limited to their bodies but emanating out, like radio beacons, mixing with other minds and energies in a bowl of consciousness soup we call humankind. But our minds contain not just our conscious thoughts but also all the conflicting emotions, desires, thoughts, and images that we have, many of which reside in our subconscious. So the energy soup of humankind as a whole can get kind of thick, which could explain why an individual's reality might not contain what that one person consciously thought of and wished for.

A number of influences are likely responsible for our experiences in the world, including our conflicting subconscious desires—the effects of swimming through the consciousness soup and other yet to be discovered influences. It seems that at this point in human development our view of the total scheme of cause and effect is limited. "You create your own reality" may ultimately be true in some sense, but at this moment in evolution it may not be a useful concept for the vast majority of people, including cancer patients.

Even though our beliefs and stressful emotions may play a role in illness, it is not because we choose them intentionally to limit us. More likely, past emotional experiences created beliefs that have depleted our immune system. This is not something a rational person would blame anyone for. It is more like an accident, where events unfolded unintentionally and with an undesired result.

Unfortunately, some people take the complicated concept of manifestation, reduce it to a belief that "we create our reality," and jump to the conclusion that we must also cause our illness. This is a chain of associations that can create deep feelings of self-blame. People fail to offer forgiveness to themselves, as they naturally would to others who engage in unintentional behaviors.

Unless you are well on your way to being a spiritual master, sage or saint, I believe the chances of being able to create health through willfully manifesting it are slim. But if you are so inclined, you should try. It is probably useful to temper this awareness with acceptance of what you are experiencing in the present moment and of your limita-tions—which includes accepting that you cannot know everything. We can work on the level we are aware of, using the tools available to us. We can heal our emotions and possibly bring relief to our immune systems, which in turn may promote physical healing.

Imagery is probably the most accessible and well-researched tech-nique that is related, at least theoretically, to the concept of manifes-tation (see "Imagery," chapter 6).

Book

David Spangler, *Everyday Miracles: The Inner Art of Manifestation* (New York: Bantam, 1996).

Edgar Cayce

Edgar Cayce (1877–1945) was a devoted Christian, who in the 1930s and '40s answered questions on a range of topics, including medical conditions, while in a trance state. He was called "the sleeping prophet" because his trances resembled sleep, and after he awoke, he never remembered what had transpired. Cayce became well known for his diagnostic ability and simple folk-cures, which were approxi-mately 90 percent successful. Doctors would routinely consult Cayce regarding hard-to-treat patients, and Cayce never charged any fees for his services.

So impressive was Cayce's work that an organization, the Associa-tion for Research and Enlightenment (A.R.E.), was established to organize and disseminate the information he channeled for those who needed it. To this day people continue to use his information to suc-cessfully treat a variety of ailments. One example is Dr. Jack Pagano of Englewood Cliffs, New Jersey, who has been able to cure psoriasis repeatedly, using Cayce's suggestions for the condition.

Cayce said their were nineteen different types of cancer, very few of which originated psychologically or karmically (having their origin in past lives). Most cancers, he said, were caused by either a physical injury or an injury brought about by wear and tear on the body because of poor care, such as a lack of proper nutrition. Cayce's cura-tive recommendations ranged from surgery to carbon ash, a substance he explained how to make and administer. In almost all cases, he recommended that people with cancer avoid the nightshade family of vegetables, which includes tomatoes, peppers, and eggplant.

The Cayce philosophy of healing is simple and unadorned: all healing comes from within, from that divine source from which all life springs. All treatments, both conventional and alternative, he said, merely attune the body to that inner source of healing and awake the divine within. The Cayce readings on cancer are available from the A.R.E.

Organization

Association for Research and Enlightenment (A.R.E.)
P.O. Box 595
Virginia Beach, VA 23451
Phone: 800-333-4499

Healers

The prominent Eastern medical view is that disease starts as, and is, a manifestation of a blockage of the natural energy flows in the body. One explanation of how healers are able to promote healing is that they have the ability to consciously move energy, to release blockages and reestablish natural energy circulation in the body. This healing work is similar to what is accomplished with a variety of energy-balancing therapies, such as acupuncture, therapeutic touch, and Reiki. Therapeutic touch and Reiki practitioners pass their hands over or hold them on the surface of the body to reestablish energy movement. Therapeutic touch and increasingly Reiki are gaining widespread acceptance, even in conventional medicine, and are being used by hospital nursing staff.

Healers have, on occasion, been responsible for documented cases of miraculous cures and spontaneous remissions. Mr. Harry Edwards (1893–1976), a famous healer of the Spiritualist Church, was responsible for hundreds of such cures. His healings and advocacy for the creation in all churches of healing sanctuaries similar to those in the Spiritualist Church created a great deal of controversy with the conservative churches in England. Healers and any other people willing to lend their healing energies gather in the healing sanctuary after services to participate in healing or prayers for those, present or absent, in need of healing. "Absent healing," or healing for those not present, takes the form of prayers and visualizations of healing for those in need. It is a free service offered by Spiritualist churches.

Healers with Edward's extraordinary talent are rare indeed. The chances of finding a person so capable of healing are about as low as of finding a true saint. It is possible, but not so likely that a sensible person would rely on it. My own experience has been that the effectiveness of the average healer is about the same as that of most subtle energy techniques. Short-term relief is common, but curative results are rare. This is not to say the practices are without benefit; they might serve an individual's healing in the larger sense of reducing stress and strengthening the immune system. Often energy is moved and the natural energy balance is restored, at least briefly. Unless underlying conditions that brought about the blockage are resolved, however, the relief is often only temporary.

Books

Harry Edwards, *A Guide to the Understanding and Practice of Spiritual Healing* (Burrows Lea, England: Healer Publishing, 1974).

Barbara Ann Brennan, *Hands of Light: A Guide to Healing Through the Human Energy Field* (New York: Bantam, 1987).

Barbara Ann Brennan, *Light Emerging: The Journey of Personal Healing* (New York: Bantam, 1993).

Dolores Krieger, Ph.D., R.N., *The Therapeutic Touch: How to Use Your Hands to Help to Heal* (New York: Simon & Schuster, 1992).

Susan Wager, M.D., and Dora Kunz, *A Doctor's Guide to Therapeutic Touch: Enhancing the Body's Energy to Promote Healing* (New York: Perigee/Putnam, 1996).

Diane Stein, *Essential Reiki: A Complete Guide to an Ancient Healing Art* (Freedom, CA: Crossing Press, 1995).

William Lee Rand, *Reiki: The Healing Touch* (Southfield, MI: Vision Publications, 1991). Available by calling 800-332-8112.

Organizations

For information, books, and referrals to Spiritualist churches near you:

National Spiritualist Association of Churches (NSAC)
13 Cottage Row
Lilydale, NY 14752
Phone: 716-595-2000

The names of people in need of healing are collected and sent to Spiritualist churches within and outside of the U.S. once each month. To obtain absent healing, send the name of the individual in need to:

NSAC Healing Center
c/o Gene Pfortmiller
3521 West Topeka Drive
Glendale, AZ 85308

Internal Wisdom

The idea that a wise and loving spiritual force, Oneness, or God is at the core of humans is very old. Many people have found that gaining access to their core energy or wisdom can provide specific information that is helpful for healing their specific illnesses. This font of wisdom can be reached through meditation, guided imagery, self-guided imagery, many psychotherapies, and many spiritual paths.

Joan Borysenko, Ph.D., described intriguing research that supports the therapeutic approach of accessing a spiritual and knowledgeable source of information within during her interview for my documentary *Cancer: Increasing Your Odds for Survival* (see interview, chapter 6). Referring to studies done in the 1970s by psychotherapist Ralph Allison, Ph.D., with people with multiple personality disorder, she observed that he found all the patients had within them a personality who claimed not to be formed at a particular moment in time like the rest of the personalities formed through instances of severe abuse. "Regardless of the religious background of the person involved, that personality would describe itself with terms like 'I am the wisdom self, I am a conduit for divine love, I am the divine spark of the person.' Often this inner self would say things like 'I have been with the person from the time before they took a body, and I will continue to be with that person until they lay their body down.'"

Communicating with this inner helper, Allison found, yielded very specific feedback about the patient's therapy and the process of integrating the disparate subpersonalities, or false selves, into a functional whole. Because this personality had such reliable information, Allison came to call it the inner-self helper. Observes Borysenko, "I think we are all a little bit like multiple personalities in that the work of a lifetime for each one of us is to let down those false selves and to come back in touch with the most true core of our being."

Many spiritually based psychotherapies have discovered the usefulness of a voice that appears to be associated with a higher power within us. It seems to be an inner helper. Whether you call it Jesus, God, the Light Within, or an angel, and whether it is real or imagined, it has demonstrated itself capable of providing useful information regarding the health of the individual. Many therapies and guided imagery exercises have been developed to assist people in communicating with this inner helper in order to obtain information helpful to their healing. One of the best therapies for this is psychosynthesis (see "Psychosynthesis" in chapter 7, also "Meditation" and "Imagery" in chapter 6).

Organization

Simonton Cancer Center
P.O. Box 890
Pacific Palisades, CA 90272
Phone: 800-459-3424
Phone: 800-338-2360 (for books and tapes)

Uses guided imagery to contact the inner healer in its approach.

Books

All by Stephen Levine:

Stephen Levine, *Guided Meditations, Explorations, and Healings* (New York: Anchor/Doubleday, 1991).

Stephen Levine, *Healing into Life and Death* (New York: Anchor/Doubleday, 1987).

Stephen Levine, *Meetings at the Edge: Dialogues with the Grieving and Dying, the Healing and the Healed* (Garden City, NY: Anchor/Doubleday, 1984).

202 CANCER: INCREASING YOUR ODDS FOR SURVIVAL

Stephen Levine, *Who Dies? An Investigation of Conscious Living and Conscious Dying* (New York: Anchor/Doubleday, 1982).

Stephen Levine, *A Year to Live: How to Live This Year as If It Were Your Last* (New York: Bell Tower, 1997).

Books and audiotapes by Steven Levine are available from:

Warm Rock Tapes
P.O. Box 100
Chamisal, NM 87525
Phone: 800-731-HEAL

Medical Astrology

"There are other things in heaven and earth . . ." observed Shakespeare, and to assume that we know all there is to know is supreme arrogance. Although my credibility is at risk, I am obligated, by my goal to be comprehensive, to include any information that may be helpful. And many people have found astrology, when practiced by a serious astrologer (not the newspaper variety), a useful tool for psychological diagnosis and counseling.

Astrology evolved at a time in history when the world and the universe were seen as a single living organism—an interconnected web of vital energies. Except for the French researcher, Michael Gauquelin, who showed that planetary patterns do coincide with some vocations, little scientific research has verified its claims.

Yet, in gifted hands, astrology can be useful. Medical astrologers specialize in helping people with medical problems overcome any psychological impediments to health by exploring possible influences such as attitudes, motives, psychological complexes, life issues, and, possibly, issues from past lives that have been carried forward. At the very least, astrological information may serve as a mirror to a person's less conscious workings. Like the *I Ching* or other tools of divination, it is believed astrological readings work because people hear in the reading what they need to hear. At its best, people report gaining valuable insight that has accelerated the psycho-spiritual growth they seek. As with other practices involving intuitional and subtle energies, good practitioners are rare.

Organization

American Federation of Astrologers
P.O. Box 22040
Tempe, AZ 85285
Phone: 602-838-1751 or 888-301-7630

Book

Dane Rudhyar, *The Astrology of Personality: A Reformulation of Astrological Concepts and Ideals in Terms of Contemporary Psychology and Philosophy* (Santa Fe, NM: Aurora Press, 1990). Reorients astrology as a tool for creative exploration of life directions and for psychological diagnosis and counseling.

Practitioner

Ingrid Naiman
P.O. Box 31007
Santa Fe, NM 87594-1007
Phone: 505-473-5797

Dr. Naiman is a well-known medical astrologer and herbalist. She currently provides only in-person consultations, but she can make referrals to other astrologers she has trained. She has written *The Astrology of Healing: Cancer* (Santa Fe, NM: Seventh Ray Press, 1988), which is fascinating although it is more useful for astrologers. Contact her for a complete list of publications and audiocassettes.

Medical Intuitives and Psychics

When most people think of psychics, they think of psychic hotlines. This misrepresents the *few* truly intuitive individuals who deserve the name. Psychics who specialize in giving medical advice, also called medical intuitives, may be helpful in gaining insight into an illness. A medical intuitive may provide information about a person's disease, psychology, and emotional blockages that need resolution.

The collaboration of Carolyn Myss, a talented medical intuitive, with C. Norman Shealy, M.D., Ph.D., the founder of the American Holistic Medical Association, has helped bring credibility to this phenomenon. With proven accuracy, Myss is able to "see" illnesses in a person's body through intuitive means and is able to help people understand the emotional, psychological, and physical developmental issues of an illness. Unfortunately, there are so few people with this rare talent, I cannot recommend you spend your time trying to find one.

If you wish to consult a psychic, be sure you have a strong personal recommendation from someone whose judgment you trust. And check the accuracy of the information you receive against your own intuition. Even good psychics are more skilled in giving insight into your personal psychology than they are at predicting the future, since knowledge of the future is highly speculative. Good psychics often avoid predicting the future, because everything is subject to change.

Personal and psychological insight into your illness, however, can be useful. Mind-body techniques like imagery and psychotherapy are potentially more accurate methods of gaining access to this type of information. Therapists are trained to help elicit such information from the client, so since it is coming from you rather than someone else, its validity is less questionable than that of psychic pronouncements. Some therapists believe that there is a source of inner healing wisdom that exists within all of us, but few people are capable of contacting it without help (see "Internal Wisdom," this chapter). Some therapies, like psychosynthesis (see "Psychosynthesis," chapter 7) are excellent at this. For an account of psychic information about cancer that was channeled in the earlier part of the century, see "Edgar Cayce" (this chapter).

Books

Caroline M. Myss, Ph.D., *Why People Don't Heal and How They Can* (New York: Harmony Books, 1997). The story, observations, and revelations of a talented medical intuitive.

Caroline M. Myss, Ph.D., and C. Norman Shealy, M.D., *The Creation of Health: The Emotional, Psychological, and Spiritual Responses That Promote Health and Healing* (New York: Three Rivers Press, 1998).

Past Lives

Some people have found that working with past lives provides another entry point into their psychology and their healing process. In this view of reality, which is held by many religions, especially Eastern ones, a person's spiritual center or soul continues after death, bringing into the next life the energetic experiences from its previous lives. In some cultures this core experience is called karma, or the lessons remaining to be learned before leaving the cycle of physical life to rejoin the oneness from which we came. Two-thirds of the world's population is said to believe they have lived before. Reincarnation was even taught by the early Christian church until it was outlawed as heresy. There are numerous substantiated cases where young children have insisted they have a different name and home and, when taken to that location, have located objects they had hidden in places they have never visited in their present lives. Also, many people through hypnosis have recalled verifiable facts of a previously living person's life—a life about which they had no prior information in this life.

Past-life therapy has become an unofficial, little-talked-about specialty in psychology that uses trance-induction techniques to regress clients to recollections of past lives. Clients often experience understanding and resolution of past- and present-life circumstances. But what if the images of past lives that people experience in trance are just products of their imaginations? One therapist pointed out to me that it was impossible to prove if recollections of past lives were real, but, real or not, the imagery produced by the client accurately symbolized some inner process and was therefore useful therapeutically. As an accurate projection of the person's subconscious, the images provided useful starting points for addressing the person's present issues. Seeing some present-day trauma symbolized in a past life can provide a safe avenue for dealing with the present trauma.

Books

Brian Weiss, M.D., *Many Lives, Many Masters* (New York: Simon & Schuster, 1988).

Roger Woolger, Ph.D., *Other Lives, Other Selves: A Jungian Psychotherapist Discovers Past Lives* (New York: Doubleday, 1987).

Prayer

Prayer is one method some people have used to contact the loving life force they call God. Prayer can be used to implore, or it can be used to align with the healing force. One double-blind experiment demonstrated that people who were being prayed for did significantly better than those in the control group who were not.

Books

Larry Dossey, M.D., *Be Careful What You Pray For... You Just Might Get It* (San Francisco, CA: HarperSanFrancisco, 1997).

Larry Dossey, M.D., *Healing Words: The Power of Prayer and the Practice of Medicine* (San Francisco, CA: HarperSanFrancisco, 1993).

Larry Dossey, M.D., *Prayer Is Good Medicine: How to Reap the Healing Benefits of Prayer* (San Francisco, CA: HarperSanFrancisco, 1996).

Agnes Mary White Sanford, *The Healing Light: The Art and Method of Spiritual Healing* (New York: Ballantine, 1990).

Spiritual Paths: *A Course in Miracles*

A Course in Miracles (ACIM) is a spiritual path that has been helpful to many people. It consists of three books: a text, a handbook for teachers, and a workbook consisting of three hundred and sixty-five lessons, one for each day of the year. The course was scribed by Helen Schucman, a Jewish psychologist who received the information from a nonphysical entity. Schucman, after doubting her sanity, sought professional advice and was found to be sane. She did nothing with the material for many years. Friends who were impressed by the profound and important lessons of the course formed A Foundation for Inner Peace and published the material.

The language used is Christian, but the framework is more Eastern and is similar to Buddhist teachings in many respects. It is often called a course in forgiveness. God is seen as totally loving and nonjudgmental. Physical reality is seen as the result of a portion of the God energy (the ego) separating from the oneness of God. This separated "Son of God" felt guilty and feared God's wrath for separating from him. Because of this, guilt and fear became an integral part of physical reality. According to *A Course in Miracles,* disease is a manifestation of fear, which arises from being alienated from our source, God. In this view, disease can be dealt with more adequately from a God-centered perspective.

Although not a path for healing disease, ACIM is a path for spiritual healing that some people have found to be helpful. *A Course in Miracles* is somewhat difficult to grasp but easy to follow and useful to those to whom it speaks. It is recommended for those who may be seeking a worthy spiritual path and spiritual understanding.

Books

Gerald Jampolsky, M.D., *Love Is Letting Go of Fear* (Berkeley, CA: Celestial Arts, 1979).

Kenneth Wapnick, Ph.D., *A Talk Given on a Course in Miracles: An Introduction,* 4th ed. (Roscoe, NY: Foundation for A Course in Miracles, 1996).

Kenneth Wapnick, Ph.D., and Gloria Wapnick, *Awaken from the Dream* (Roscoe, NY: Foundation for A Course in Miracles, 1995).

Organizations

Foundation for Inner Peace
P.O. Box 598
Mill Valley, CA 94942
Phone: 415-388-2060

Publisher of *A Course in Miracles* (1975, 1985) and resource for additional information.

Foundation for A Course in Miracles
1275 Tennanah Lake Road
Roscoe, NY 12776
Phone: 607-498-4116

Offers related courses, workshops, books, and tapes.

Spiritual Paths: Pathwork

John Pierrakos, M.D., a psychiatrist and cofounder of the psychotherapy called bioenergetics (see "Bioenergetics," chapter 7), was married to Eva Pierrakos, a medium or channel. Channels have existed throughout most of recorded history in many cultures, including ancient Greece, where they were known as oracles. Channels, or mediums, usually go into a trance state in which they are capable of allowing external, nonphysical, hopefully prophetic sources of wisdom to communicate through them.

When Eva Pierrakos began receiving channeled information, her psychiatrist husband, who could find nothing psychologically wrong with his wife, soon became amazed at the psychological depth with which the "guide," who spoke through his wife, answered his questions. The guide delivered, through Eva, two hundred and fifty-eight lectures on the nature of psychological and spiritual reality and outlined a path for spiritual development. This spiritual development process came to be called the Pathwork.

The Pathwork is not for everyone. It is psychologically deep and challenging. Regardless of whether or not you believe in channeling, the material is profound and useful. Its goal is to achieve an understanding and experience of the enlightened, loving core, or God within, which is believed to be at the center of all people. It is especially of interest for those wanting a balanced psychological and spiritual path.

Books

Eva Pierrakos, *The Path of Self-Transformation* (New York: Bantam, 1990). Excellent summary of the Pathwork lectures.

Susan Thesenga, *The Undefended Self: Living the Pathwork of Spiritual Wholeness,* 2d ed. (Madison, VA: Pathwork Press, 1994).

Organization

Phoenicia Pathwork Center
P.O. Box 66
Phoenicia, NY 12464
Phone: 914-688-2211

Sells individual guide lectures on specific topics and offers courses and workshops related to the Pathwork.

Chapter Resources

Books

Joan Borysenko, Ph.D., *Guilt Is the Teacher, Love Is the Lesson* (New York: Warner Books, 1990). One of the best overviews of psychospirituality. Highly recommended.

Deepak Chopra, M.D., *Quantum Healing: Exploring the Frontiers of Mind/Body Medicine* (New York: Bantam, 1989).

Larry Dossey, M.D., *Recovering the Soul: A Scientific and Spiritual Search* (New York: Bantam, 1989).

Bernie S. Siegel, M.D., *How to Live Between Office Visits: A Guide to Life, Love and Health* (New York: HarperCollins, 1993).

Bernie S. Siegel, M.D., *Love, Medicine, & Miracles: Lessons Learned About Self-Healing from a Surgeon's Experience with Exceptional Patients* (New York: Harper & Row, 1986).

Bernie S. Siegel, M.D., *Peace, Love, & Healing: Bodymind Communication and the Path to Self-Healing: An Exploration* (New York: Harper & Row, 1989).

Tapes

Dr. Bernie Siegel's videotapes are available from:

Mystic Five Video
Phone: 1-800-861-3296

Touchstar
Phone: 1-800-861-3296

Dr. Siegel's audiotapes are available from:

Hay House
Phone: 800-654-5126

Organization

Mind/Body Health Sciences, Inc.
393 Dixon Road
Boulder, CO 80302
Phone: 303-440-8460

This is Joan Borysenko's organization; it offers the *Circles of Healing Newsletter.*

Practitioners

Joan Borysenko, Ph.D. (see "Organizations," above). Available for speaking engagements.

Bernie Siegel, M.D.
Fax: 203-387-8355
Email: bugsysiegel@compuserve.com

Available for speaking engagements.

Interview with
Bernie Siegel, M.D.

on the Paradox of Illness and Healing, Being Able to Say No, Loving Yourself, and Spirituality

Dr. Bernie Siegel, who is now retired from general and pediatric surgery, founded Exceptional Cancer Patients (ECaP) in 1978. ECaP is based on "carefrontation," a safe, loving, therapeutic confrontation that facilitates personal lifestyle changes, personal empowerment, and healing of the individual's life. The physical, spiritual, and psychological benefits that follow such changes led to his desire to make each person aware of his or her own healing potential. He is the author of *Love, Medicine & Miracles: Lessons Learned About Self-Healing from a Surgeon's Experience with Exceptional Patients; Peace, Love & Healing: Bodymind Communication and the Path to Self-Healing: An Exploration*; and *How to Live Between Office Visits: A Guide to Life, Love and Health.* More than any other person, he has brought to popular attention evidence, research, and anecdotes of the psychological and spiritual aspects of healing. He is alive with excitement about the information he has discovered.

Let's start by talking about how the Simonton workshop got you started, and how you were amazed that this information was accepted as old hat in some circles.

When I began to get interested in this whole mind-body area, I didn't have any training, and that is mostly because medicine doesn't train you in this area. I was very happy to see the Simonton book come out, *Getting Well Again*. When [the Simontons] came to a nearby community, I saw that flyer and I thought, wow, every doctor will want to go!

It is incredible to me that there was not one single oncologist from the whole state. Even if the oncologists didn't believe, at least they could see what people were saying. The thing that opened me most [about the Simontons] was that you could sit and share with your patients in a different way—no desk interceding—and they could really talk to you about their experiences.

And then two important things happened to me. One was my own patient saying, "I need to know how to live between office visits." That was something that never occurred to me—again, you don't have a course in medical school teaching you how to help people live. The other was the power of the guided imagery that Carl [Simonton] got up to do. At first it sounded like nonsense, so I wasn't even going to close my eyes or bother to participate; but, since I was sitting very close to him in the second row, I knew he would look at me, and I didn't have the courage to sit there with my eyes open. I admire lots of people who sit there and stare back at you during imagery; that takes a lot of courage. I also know that it can be happening for them even with their eyes open. At any rate, I said, I'll close my eyes so he won't be bothered and won't look at me. And when I closed my eyes, being an artist and a very visual person, some incredible things happened for me, and that changed me. Because now, you see, it wasn't something somebody lectured about, it was something that *happened* to me.

And so I went back really enthused. I recorded all my feelings after [the workshops]. You could hear the change in me on the tapes because of the experience I had, meeting an inner guide and having all those things happen. I [began to] put together what I thought of *as a little course to teach people how to live between visits*. And so we started, in the fall of '78, planning to have eight sessions; and of course, thirteen years later we are still running, because once you begin to learn how hard living is, you are never going to teach anybody in two months how to deal with every possible problem that life will ever bring them.

I also, at that point, saw what happened when you brought these techniques into people's lives. I saw people doing all these things: straightening their lives out and then not dying when they were supposed to, responding to therapy or, even if they weren't getting therapy, responding to lifestyle changes. And that is when I began to write articles thinking, "I shouldn't keep this a secret; this is wonderful." I mailed them out to all the medical journals, and they came back saying, "This is interesting but inappropriate for our journal"—I just wish I had saved all these letters—and then I mailed them to where I thought it would be appropriate, and they came back saying, "This is appropriate but not interesting."

That's when I was awakened to the fact that there were an incredible number of people out there who were aware of what I had learned—psychologists, social workers, Jungian therapists, hypnotherapists—who had been doing this for years, and I was mad. Why wasn't it taught to me as a physician? Why didn't they tell me to use these techniques to help people?

So I just really worked at improving and learning and reading incredible amounts about these areas, and [I kept] coming across things that were astonishing to me, and again they made me angry. I still get angry: six decades have gone by since Carl Jung interpreted a dream and made a physical diagnosis, and yet I have run into probably fewer than six students who have ever been told this, and I am talking about thousands of medical students.

There seems to be a fine line between the idea that we manifest our reality and the idea that we are to blame for it. You have been accused of encouraging people to take a look at their participation in their illnesses, causing them to blame themselves. What are you really saying, and how is blame avoided?

The biggest problem we run into in this area is children [being] raised to feel inadequate, guilty, blameful, shameful—it is a horror—and when you ask people to just make an effort to get well, they are afraid to because they could do it wrong or fail at it. Unfortunately, a lot of people carry this to an extreme: that if anything is wrong with you, you did something wrong.

Too many people look at what you need to change as, "What did I do wrong?" One medical student's wife looked at [it instead] as "the process of transformation." She said, "I didn't feel I did anything wrong, but the cancer led me to more transformation and more growth."

We can distort or misinterpret that message. When I [ask], "How can you benefit from or why do you need an illness?" if the answer is "I don't," then [I] go on to the next question. But if [the patient] sits there for three days thinking, "What did I do wrong, and did I cause this?" and he is telling me, "I'm guilty," then my [question] is: "Why do you feel guilty when somebody else just finished the book [*Love, Medicine & Miracles*] and said, "I'm inspired?" It gets back to our upbringing—that we see in those pages what our parents did to us and what our religions did to us. Plenty of people out there are absolutely sure they are being punished, and so they are not supposed to get well or get their child well because God has caught up with them for the terrible things they have done.

All this needs to be dealt with, but isn't dealt with in medical school. Nobody ever told me that somebody might want to be operated on in order to be punished for their sins. So, those are things I had to learn about people by asking the right questions [about] what was happening in their lives and letting them express their story.

How is it possible that love heals, and what role can the spiritual play in healing a cancer?

If feelings are chemical, my simple way of always making these things scientific [is by] talking "neuropeptides." I think the healthiest feeling is love, unconditional love, giving with no expectations. Now, [take] volunteers, for instance. Some studies have been done: they volunteer two hours a week to help people they are not related to, they stay healthier, and some of them, when examined after the volunteer work, were physically better.

What you are seeing are the changes that occur when you are contributing to the world. Carl Menninger used the word *cure* where I would put *heal*, but he said love cures two people—the person who gives it and the person who receives it. My homework question is, "How can you be happy for the rest of your life? You realize that that is doing for others out of love."

The other side of the coin [is being able to say no]. This gets to be confusing for a lot of people; they say that if you are loving, how can you get angry, how can you say no? I say, wait a minute, if somebody steps on your foot, can't you say, "You're stepping on my foot"? Somebody hangs a sign on your door in the hospital that [says] you're a "lymphoma," can't you take that off and say, "No, I'm a human being, not a lymphoma"? So, it's okay—it doesn't mean you're not a lover. So, it's asserting yourself.

George Solomon, a psychiatrist, asks one question of people with AIDS. He said it predicts long-term survival. [He asks,] "Would you do a favor for a friend that you don't want to do?" Most people conveniently leave out the last part or [don't] see it: you don't want to do something. But the majority of people say yes. They are not likely to be long-term survivors.

So, what I am asking is "How do you want to love the world tomorrow?" If my way of loving the world doesn't include what you're asking of me, then I have a right to say no. Or if I really love what you have asked of me, then the whole question changes, then I am glad to drop my plans and rush off to help you because I will come home flying high, feeling real good, and you don't ever have to say thanks. This is my way of serving the world—and that is what we are really here for.

So, I get ultimately to the point of asking people: "How can you die laughing, and what is your life about?" And they begin to understand [that] if you are here to serve, then you feel good. We all need people, and everybody is in pain, so don't be worried, the person next to you has the same troubles you have. Then I think you begin to see what love is about. Most of us are brought up on conditional love: I give you two hours of my love, you owe me two hours of your love, and if you only give me ninety minutes then I resent you. And you don't get invited to my daughter's wedding, and then you're mad at me, and it goes on and on.

When you love unconditionally, a lot of wonderful things begin to happen because it comes back. I always look back at what has been manifested from my work when I decided to help twelve patients. Look what happened to me. I didn't plan to write a book, I didn't plan to talk to anybody, I was just going to meet a couple hours a week and talk to my patients. But I think once you begin to help people live, it is incredible how those ripples go out, and the word gets around, and more people start showing up, and they want help living. That is really the biggest problem.

The other question I ask is, "Is life fair?" The majority of every single group I ever talked to says no. That includes doctors, wellness conferences, you name it. And my comment always is, "Then why are you having a wellness conference? You should have an unwellness conference." And doctors—I said to the Yale Medical School graduating class, "If life isn't fair, don't you dare go out there and get people to live longer. Do you want them to suffer more?" They looked at me with this puzzled expression. See, nobody has ever brought that up to them. If life is difficult, why make people live longer?

One classical example—and I never make up these stories—a lady said, "I took all my pills, lay down in bed to commit suicide, and the phone rang." To me that is the height of absurdity—you're trying to die and the phone is ringing. What do you do? Most audiences roar because they know the dilemma. They know damn well they would get up off the bed, go to the phone, pick it up, and say, "Yes?" And what she said was, "On the way to the phone I realized, I don't have to kill myself, I just have to stop answering the telephone!" So it saved her life. This is why, when people feel out of control, not living their lives, love doesn't come into it and they do get sicker and die faster.

But the love and the spirituality that comes with it when God is a resource, not a punisher—. Then wonderful things happen for those people. And it is physiologic; none of this is what I would call mystical. I call it all scientific—that a belief in God keeps your blood pressure lower. Is that God doing it? No, it's your peace, which comes with that, and with the love and all the things that go into it. And you see this whether it's cancer, AIDS, a prisoner in a concentration camp, [someone] lost in a life raft. When you talk to survivors of life's catastrophes, they all sound alike. And that's why I think, let's spread the word around so that those of us who choose to live [can] keep confronting the difficulties. [I remember] Joseph Campbell saying that the great gurus of the world are always the ones who know how to find joy in the sorrow. And that's what I know life is about, and why I spend a good deal of time laughing as well as hurting—because of a lot of lovely people I know.

And my mortality—let me just give you an example: I know that I am going to die, that is why I enjoy life. [I had] a hundred people sitting in front of [me] with cancer, and I read them a letter I got that day, and it said, "young doctor just beginning her practice got stung by a bee and is dead in three days from anaphylactic shock." That is reality. A young doctor calls me—student who works with me—he fell off a cliff, fractured his back, and is now in a cast for three months; lucky he is not paralyzed. And another student who is now a doctor who was in an auto accident *is* paralyzed. To me that is reality. I know damn well that something could happen to me on the way home, and therefore I really choose life in this moment and live that way. And that is what I am trying to get people to do. [When you live life this way] God becomes a resource not a punisher.

What is your personal belief about the nature of that love: is it something that lives inside of all people?

To me the definition of God is creative intelligent energy. You can't, I think, be a scientist without being filled with awe and wonder. I always talk about ice and Band-Aids as proof of God's existence, because ice is the only substance that becomes lighter than the liquid when you freeze it; no other liquid does that. Every other liquid when frozen becomes denser and sinks. How come ice doesn't do that? If you want to keep this planet alive, you better keep the ice on top. So somebody [intelligent] had to decide to keep the ice on top or else we'd kill everything. And Band-Aids—I really laugh, because every time I cut my finger or get a blister, I get very happy because I put a Band-Aid [on it], and I take it off a week later and there is nothing there. And I think, "Wow, that is exciting. That shows me that there is creative intelligence in me that knows how to heal—no directions, no book, no instructions." And that is God for me, this wonderful intelligence.

Now, since we all come from that, we are a unit. So I think, in a sense, the love is the love of ourselves as well as our participating in each other. We are all one, and that is part of the struggle that is going on in this world right now. So I really see helping heal the individual as also preserving the planet. I don't think you can separate them. Someone who grows up loved and believing in that unity is going to treat this planet a lot differently than those who don't.

And I think our mechanistic professions, our civilization—which is really more uncivilized—has separated us from nature. When I go out in the morning and listen to the sounds of nature, I become very spiritual. You go out in the city in the middle of day, you're not very spiritual, you do not get connected back to the earth again. Native Americans were [spiritual] because they were out there as part of the earth. When they make a decision for seven generations from today, they are not kidding; they know what they can do. But we don't say, "Let's think about it, before we pass this law, what it will do to seven generations." We are thinking about next week and next month, the budget and how are we going to get through the year—and that's sad. That affects us at all levels. My hope is that the pain and the cost of disease is going to pressure us back to wellness and understanding all these things we are talking about, and I think that is slowly beginning to happen.

Could you do me a favor and talk about why it is important for people to love themselves, what that brings to them?

If you talk about being well, it is being empowered: making your choices, [doing] all the things that, when you love yourself, develop self-esteem. You keep your power. You are not afraid to deal with the medical profession or family. You are not afraid to make choices. There may be a point where you say, "No, I don't want that" or "That is enough" or "Yes, I will do this," even if your family says, "That's terrible." One young man I was dealing with—his father said, "There are three good reasons you shouldn't die: your mother, me, and you." I said, "One out of three is right—you—but don't go through it for them." His friends also drove him to the cemetery and said, "We don't want you dead and here." I said, "That's easy. Tell your friends they're to have chemotherapy, radiation, and a bone marrow transplant with you." He smiled and liked that idea.

That's why you need the self-esteem, self-worth, self-love, so you can say to your friends, "Hey, that's my choice. I don't go through it for you, because, otherwise, I will know how to punish my friends. I will have so many side effects they will say, 'Gee, we're sorry. Quit!'"

So this boy's friends have eased up on him. They realized what they did was wrong. When you take charge of your life, there may be sadness and grief and sick or dying, but it's your life and you are living it now.

How do you begin loving yourself?

One of the questions I'm often asked is how I can help [people who don't love themselves], and my answer is that I keep loving them. So if you come to my office fifty pounds overweight, haven't bathed in a year, drug addicted, what am I going to do with you? Especially when you say, "Can I hug you?" I do hug you, and I do say that I will see you next week, no matter how obnoxious you are, no matter how much you don't listen to me. I will set some rules—there is discipline, meaning that if you do certain things I may say, "Then our relationship has ended." One day you come in and say, "I took a bath, and I'm getting a job," and I didn't say to take a bath or get a job. Why? Because I have faith in you and believe in you. I even find that from letters. I didn't change their life, I wrote them a letter, but that letter! Coming from the authority figure who has written a book, [they say,] "If he wrote to me I must be worth something!" That helps, and that is like reparenting.

There are people who have said, "I stood in front of a mirror naked to find something lovable about myself, and I picked out my hair or my smile or my skin." God, that's work to do that every day— keeping a journal to pour out the feelings, getting the pain out, going to a group, whether it is for your alcoholism, your drug addiction, your cancer, your AIDS, whatever—to sit down and say, "Okay, I have got to talk about my life." A friend of mine, Susan Duffy—I always cite her because her whole family committed suicide and wanted her to, but she didn't—she said, "I grew up with a message, 'Die, kid, die.'" She said, "I lived in a prison. I didn't have a choice who my parents were, but one day I decided to let love into my prison, and it changed every negative item in it." She got to that point partly because I listened to her—and that is the key for every therapist and every family member: listen, listen. When I listened to her for a long enough time, she had dumped her garbage out, so love could come in. A computer friend of mine says, "If you put garbage in, you get garbage out, and if you put garbage out, love comes in." I would say, Let that person put the garbage out, and someday they will say, "I feel empty." Let some love in, don't pick up more garbage.

Yet, there are people who love picking up garbage and keep complaining that it is their pattern. I have met people who just love being sick, and I just keep loving them. That's okay, I am not going to get mad at them. The ones who are really hurting, they don't want to keep that up, and they let the love in and the change happens—not because I had answers, but because I had ears to listen to them with.

If you had one message to give cancer patients, what would it be?

The one that I noticed this week as I was reading Joseph Campbell was, Don't try to solve the problem with the mystery. As physicians, [we try] that mechanistic approach: how do we cure this disease? Gets back to Jung talking about the story of your life, the metaphor and the mystery with your life. Live the mystery.

The other [message] is from Saroyan, who said love is immortal and makes all things immortal, and Thornton Wilder, who said there is a land of the living and a land of the dead, and if the bridge is love we will all survive. Meaning: if you want to be immortal, love somebody; then a part of you lives forever.

How to die laughing on a practical level: I think there are two things involved. One is understanding what life is about and why you are here and what you are here to accomplish. If you do that, which really relates to relationships and love, then you can die with a smile. It doesn't mean you are not sad. The other is that you've got to live life in a childlike way so that when you turn to all your loved ones, who are sitting around your bed as you are trying to die, and say to them, "Would you do something and tell some anecdotes about my life—what you remember about me?" they will have some really good stories to tell. And you will lie back beaming about the craziness and the fun that you had and what you did with your kids and a whole host of other things, and you will die with a smile on your face, and they will be left feeling a hell of a lot better. And I can say, on a practical level, that is how my father died at three in the afternoon on Sunday, surrounded by his loved ones, with my mother telling stories that had us roaring. Even to the point of some of the people in the hospital room being embarrassed that they were laughing. Everyone sort of realized, "We are in a hospital—what are we doing laughing? This is fun! There is nothing wrong with laughing here!" It is just a beautiful moment when those kinds of things happen.

[All interviews have been edited for length and clarity.]

Dr. Bernie Siegel can be contacted for speaking engagements at
Fax: 203-387-8355
Email: bugsyesiegel@compuserve.com

His videotapes are available from
Mystic Five Video: 800-861-3296

and his audiotapes are available from
Hay House: 800-654-5126.

9

Cancer and Mortality

This chapter is for people who are dying of cancer and those who love and care for them. The information and resources here can help prepare for the last stages of life. During this time, people have concerns about pain management, legal issues, and the emotional challenges of communicating, letting go of life, and grieving.

There is a point when the denial of death tends to drop away. Sometimes it is when the body has been compromised beyond the point of no return and treatment has no effect. Sometimes the acceptance that a person is dying does not occur until the very end.

Cindy's desire to live and my commitment to help her in any way possible may have created denial about her dying. Admitting that Cindy was dying did not seem to further her quest for life. Yet who is to judge when it is time to let go of the struggle to live? According to Stephen Levine, author of many excellent books on death and dying, it is up to the patient. Cindy wanted to continue to fight for her life. If this was denial, then it was her choice to be in denial and die fighting. It was my job to help her do whatever she wanted.

For the first six months after Cindy died, I cried and stumbled around in a state of shock. I started working on the documentary for which this guide was written because I knew that I could help others and because working on such a project would help me heal. I avoided reading about death and dying, probably for the same reason many people avoid the concept of death: I didn't want to be reminded of Cindy's dying; I thought it would create more pain. It wasn't until I had to read *Who Dies? An Investigation of Conscious Living and Conscious Dying* (New York: Anchor/Doubleday, 1982) to prepare for interviewing its author, Stephen Levine, that I realized how I wrong I was. I wish I had read his books sooner. His words helped me heal more than anything else I had done. His writings transformed my relationship to death, and to Cindy's dying, by exposing me to many truths about death that I simply had not learned.

It is a fact of life that everyone dies. Yet, as a culture, we don't want to talk about death. It scares us. It reminds us that we, too, will die someday. Death is perhaps more difficult when it occurs sooner than expected or is part of a painful degenerative process. While this project is about helping people survive, it is an unfortunate reality that about 50 percent of people diagnosed with cancer die within five years. It would be unfair to leave the families who are faced with the devastating experience of terminal cancer without information on how to help a loved one who is dying and how to help themselves survive that loss.

Communicating

Most people have difficulty communicating with someone who may be dying; they don't know what to say. Death is foreign and frightening to most of us. In my experience, it is most important just to be there, present and ready to listen. If you wish to do more, you can ask the person what they want to talk about, or you can learn to ask questions such as, "What was the best period of your life?" or "What was the best thing you ever did?" These and other questions can be found in an excellent chapter entitled, "The Person Who Is Dying," in Lawrence LeShan's book, *Cancer as a Turning Point: A Handbook for People with Cancer, Their Families, and Health Professionals* (New York: Dutton/Penguin, 1989).

Remember not to force anyone to talk about either their life or their death. Look for openings. Tell them that you would like to hear their story; offer them the opportunity to talk about their life. Be ready and willing to listen to their fears about the end of life and any stories they wish to tell.

Some family members have a preconceived image of what the death experience should be like. It can be helpful to discuss such preconceptions with family members or a counselor in order to let go of them, and become more open and receptive to the dying person's experiences, wishes, and needs.

It is also important to be aware that unconscious people often can hear what is being said in the room and will remember it upon awaking. Visitors need to assume the patient is hearing everything, even if they are unconscious.

Helpful activities include: touch; prayer; playing music favored by the patient; expressions of love (verbal and written); reading stories, news, poetry, or other things enjoyed by the patient; giving flowers; seeing friends; and saying good-bye.

Books

Books by Steven Levine (see "Chapter Resources" at the end of this chapter).

Family Response

Terminal diagnoses are often hidden from the dying. This denies the dying person the right to deal with the end of her life. It can be helpful for family members to discuss among themselves their feelings about the diagnosis and the imminent loss of their loved one. Sometimes the dying person conveys her desire to talk about death and related topics. If family members are uncomfortable and avoid these conversations, it is important for the family to at least offer the dying person someone to talk with who is trained and compassionate (see "Helpers," in this chapter).

Fear of Death

Often people have a fearful concept of what happens after death, and they may fear the unknown. It is important to allow the dying person opportunities to verbalize fears and concerns. Imposing your own religious or spiritual beliefs is inappropriate. You may ask questions, such as: "Are you afraid of death?" and "What do you think will happen?" Trained counselors are helpful if family members feel unable to discuss the fear of death.

Books

Raymond A. Moody, M.D., *The Light Beyond* (New York: Bantam, 1989). Anecdotal accounts of life after death.

Kenneth Ring, *Healing Toward Omega: In Search of the Meaning of the Near-Death Experience* (New York: William Morrow, 1985).

Helpers

If the family is uncomfortable talking with the cancer patient about death, they may wish to consult with the family's clergy. Hospitals often, but not always, have a pastoral services department, which will assign someone to assist you. You may need to request that the hospital appoint a social worker, pastoral counselor, or chaplain who can help. Some helpers are specifically trained in dealing with dying patients and their families, and some are not. If the nursing staff is not responsive to your request, find out if there is a patient services department, and ask for their assistance.

Hospices usually have counselors who are available to work with people on an outpatient basis, sometimes free of charge.

People trained to help during this emotionally intense time can provide tremendous comfort. With the assistance of such helpers, all people involved have the opportunity to make peace with their relationships and with the dying process.

Pain Management

Pain management has progressed to the point that, in most cases, the patient can be pain-free and still able to communicate. If the patient or the family has any concerns, request that a consultation be arranged with a pain management specialist. As the course of the illness progresses, patients may need to decide if they want to be pain-free or able to communicate.

Books

Susan S. Lang and Richard B. Pett. *You Don't Have to Suffer: A Complete Guide to Relieving Pain for Patients and Their Families* (New York: Oxford University Press, 1994).

Pamela J. Haylock, R.N., and Carol P. Curtiss, R.N., *Cancer Doesn't Have to Hurt: How to Conquer the Pain Caused by Cancer and Cancer Treatment* (Alameda, CA: Hunter House, 1997).

Advance Directives

Advance directives provide patients with an opportunity to direct caregivers when they are no longer able to act on their own behalf, such as when they are incapacitated by disease or near death. An advance directive legally protects people's wishes about medical treatment when they can no longer communicate for themselves. This includes decisions about their health care and any steps they would like, or would not like, to be taken to prolong life if they are dying.

Information regarding advance directives is usually provided to the patient by the hospital, and time should be taken to read and respond to them. Advance directives can be spoken but usually they are written in a legal form. They differ from state to state but usually consist of some type of signed "living will" that provides written instructions regarding the measures you do and don't want taken to keep you alive. Other advance directives include granting a family member or friend power of attorney and designating someone as your "health care agent" for health care decisions. The power of attorney is a legal document that can include health care decisions; it gives someone else the right to make, and sign for, health-related decisions when the patient is no longer able to.

Fear often prevents family members from discussing these decisions. Sometimes there is the unconscious feeling that, by avoiding these issues, they can somehow avoid the loved one's death and stave off the inevitable. Unfortunately, energy that could be put to better use for the dying person is consumed by this denial.

Booklet

Shape Your Health Care Future with Health Care Advance Directives. Includes forms and instructions on preparing your own advance directives. Available free by writing to:

American Association of Retired Persons
Programs Division, Health Advocacy Services Fulfillment
601 E Street, NW

Washington, DC 20049
Phone: 202-434-2277

Organization

Choice in Dying
475 Riverside Drive, Room 1852
New York, NY 10015
Phone: 800-989-WILL (800-989-9455), also 202-338-9790

Provides counseling for individuals regarding preparing and using advance directives, such as a living will, and powers of attorney for health care.

Letting Go

Denial is a common and natural reaction to the possibility of death, both in terminal patients and their loved ones. The thought of death stirs up powerful emotions that compel some to deny that the person, or oneself, is dying.

Sometimes family members or even hospice workers wish to help the dying person have a "good death"; to complete unfinished business, say good-byes, and find meaning in their life. This requires the end of denial, and in many cases the dying person is not ready or does not want to give up their denial. There is no need to force this process. Whatever the dying person wants is what is right. If a person wishes to deny to the end of his life that he is dying, as Stephen Levine asks, "Who are you to take away his denial?" It is his dying time. Whatever is comfortable for him should be accepted.

Sooner or latter denial fades and the reality of death becomes obvious: it becomes "undeniable." Letting go entails shifting from the fighting mode, where one is seeking medical care that is designed to cure, to an acceptance that one is dying; this is also referred to as the dying mode. At this time people often enter a period of fear and despair. This is when requests for suicide or assisted suicide are common.

Letting go leads to acceptance that the person is dying and to the tasks associated with the dying mode. These include activities like healing relationships, finding meaning in one's life, and preparing for death (see also "Unfinished Business," this chapter).

Spirituality can also be very important when someone is shifting from fighting a disease to accepting that they are going to die. Many people identify very strongly with the role that they played in their life; for example, that they were providers for their family, a mother, or an executive. A person's spiritual beliefs can be instrumental in developing a larger vision of themselves, that who they are is more than what they did, and is more than the physical body. As Meg Spinella, M.Ed., a hospice chaplain who works with the dying and their families, said in her interview for the documentary:

> When that role falls away and they no longer fulfill that role it can be a time of confusion for them as to who am I if I'm not that? It is helpful for them spiritually to work with a soul worker or chaplain or whoever they happen to be connected with to develop this larger vision of themselves, so they understand that who they are, in a larger sense, will go on.

It is important to remember that while all these things—like healing relationships and preparing for death—sound good on paper, they may not be so easy to do. The point is for all involved to do their best with love and forgiveness for others and for themselves. Death seldom happens under ideal circumstances, but in the words of a wise old master, it is completely safe.

Suicide

Suicidal thoughts are common among seriously ill patients and should be taken seriously. Thoughts of suicide or assisted suicide can occur in response to the fear and despair experienced by many people after they accept that they are dying. The fear is often about having a physically and/or emotionally painful death. If the dying person can get connected to hospice services (see "Hospice/Choosing Where to Die," this chapter), then hospice workers will tell you that almost universally the desire for suicide will disappear. In hospice their pain management needs are taken very seriously, and in 98 percent of the cases their pain can be managed. Emotional and psychological needs are addressed through the services of a social worker, a chaplain, an aide, or a nurse. If you are not able to obtain hospice care, then make sure that those responsible for pain management are doing their job, and use whatever resources are available to help address emotional issues.

Another major impetus behind suicidal thoughts, in addition to inadequate pain management, is the concern that "no one really wants to care for me." Sometimes this is voiced as "no one should have to take care of me." The patient needs to hear the authentic willingness on the part of family members to provide or obtain the needed care, using hospice, in-home, or institutional care. If the family becomes resentful of the patient's need for care and attention, hospital social workers, chaplains, pastoral counselors, or hospice workers are trained to work with you to resolve your issues, but you must be willing to share your feelings about the situation (see "Helpers," this chapter).

Unfinished Business

Unfinished business refers to topics that are helpful for the dying person to address in order to achieve a peaceful resolution to her life. Three common areas of unfinished business are:

1. Legal: wills, estate plans, location of deeds, and valuables; also health-care-related legalities (see "Advance Directives," this chapter).

2. Familial. What does the patient have to do to make peace with her life and the people she loves? The dying person often naturally may seek to resolve unexpressed feelings of regret, triumph, resentment, forgiveness, and love (see "Helpers," this chapter).

3. Spiritual: What previously unexplored questions about the meaning of life, God, and what happens next are surfacing now? (See "Helpers," "Fear of Death," this chapter).

Hospice/Choosing Where to Die

There are four choices of where to die: a hospice, a nursing home, a hospital room, or at home. Some hospice services and programs offer professional care and comfort to the patient and family both in institutions and at home.

Patients often prefer dying at home, in familiar surroundings. This is not always possible. The level of care required, and the physical and spiritual limitations of the individual caregivers, may eliminate this option. People shouldn't feel guilty about not caring for their loved ones at home. It can be worse to have a sick person at home whose level of care causes resentment than to leave the caretaking to others; and sometimes family members need to stay in their family roles and not become health care providers.

Hospice is a health care facility specifically designed to meet the needs of families and patients dealing with the end of life. One phrase used to describe hospice is, "When science can no longer add days to life, more life will be added to each day." If you are unable to die at home, hospice is an excellent alternative. Hospice workers are specially trained, competent, and very kind. They are available to work with families to help care for the dying person in his or her home. Hospitals are beginning to offer hospice care within their institutions. If you have a choice, visit both. Home care agencies may also have hospice programs that provide services to patients in their homes or in health care centers.

Organizations

National Hospice Organization (NHO)
1901 N. Moore Street, Suite 901
Arlington, VA 22209
Phone: 800-658-8898 or 703-243-5900
Website: www.nho.org

A resource for hospice professionals, volunteers, and the general public for terminally ill patients and their families.

Hospicelink
Phone: 800-331-1620

Offers a directory of U.S. and Canadian hospice services.

Grieving

The cancer patient may be grieving the impending loss of her or his life, and the family members are grieving their loss of the dying person. The feelings of loss, sorrow, and hurt can be overwhelming and debilitating. Yet, the important process of grieving allows the release of loss by acknowledging and experiencing these feelings.

Many people will avoid or postpone experiencing their grief. Those who do not release their grief often endure the effects of unreleased emotions for years. This can lead to depression, even incapacitation. I remember a news story, years ago, about an English psychotherapist and his shocking approach to treating people incapacitated by grief after the loss of a loved one. These people were rendered totally dysfunctional, to the point of inaction, by grief and depression. The therapist's methods were controversial because of his seemingly unkind, "confrontational" approach. Essentially he coerced his patients to experience their suppressed feelings regarding the loss of their love. Not so remarkably, his clients cried a great deal and became functional, normal, even happy people once again.

Books

Books by Stephen Levine (see "Chapter Resources," below).

Stuart Zelman, M.D., and David Bognar, *Human Operators Manual: How Feelings Work: A Psychological Primer* (Hartford, CT: n.p., 1991). Contains information on how to regain the ability to release feelings. Available from the authors for $10.95 at P.O. Box 8241, Manchester, CT 06040, phone: 888-307-4482, or on their website: www.cancersurvival.com.

Website

GriefNet: griefnet.org. Provides support and access to grief-related resources on the Internet.

Chapter Resources

Books

I highly recommend any of Stephen Levine's books:

Stephen Levine, *Guided Meditations, Explorations, and Healings* (New York: Anchor/Doubleday, 1991).

Stephen Levine, *Healing into Life and Death* (New York: Anchor/Doubleday, 1987).

Stephen Levine, *Meetings at the Edge: Dialogues with the Grieving and Dying, the Healing and the Healed* (Garden City, NY: Anchor/Doubleday, 1984).

Stephen Levine, *Who Dies? An Investigation of Conscious Living and Conscious Dying* (New York: Anchor/Doubleday, 1982).

Stephen Levine, *A Year to Live: How to Live This Year as If It Were Your Last* (New York: Bell Tower, 1997).

Books and audiotapes by Steven Levine are available from:

Warm Rock Tapes
P.O. Box 100
Chamisal, NM 87525
Phone: 800-731-HEAL

Healing/Dying: An Interview with Stephen Levine. Videotape of Steven Levine's interview; covers questions related to healing and dying. Excellent. Available from: New Way Productions, P.O. Box 8241, Manchester, CT 06040, for $33.95. Call 888-307-4482 or order at their website, www.cancersurvival.com.

Books on Caring for the Dying

Maggie Callanan and Patricia Kelley, *Final Gifts: Understanding the Special Awareness, Needs, and Communications of the Dying* (New York: Bantam, 1997).

Timothy E. Quill, M.D., *A Midwife Through the Dying Process: Stories of Healing and Hard Choices at the End of Life* (Baltimore, MD: Johns Hopkins University Press, 1996).

Websites

Bereavement and Hospice Support Netline: www.ubalt.edu/www/bereavement

National Public Radio—End of Life: www.npr.org/programs/death

Interview with Stephen Levine

on Healing the Heart, Dealing with Death, Integrating Psychology and Spirituality, Accepting Pain, and Grieving

Stephen Levine is a Buddhist, philosopher, healer, and, with his wife, an internationally recognized teacher on issues of death and dying. His writings often include guided meditations for the healing of illness, grief, heavy emotional states, and sexual abuse and for preparing for death. He cowrote *Grist for the Mill* with Ram Dass and *Healing into Life and Death* and *Who Dies? An Investigation of Conscious Living and Conscious Dying* with Ondrea Levine. He has taught meditation in the California prison system and led workshops with Elizabeth Kübler-Ross, and, while working with the terminally ill, he began to formulate his concepts of healing. His other works include *A Year to Live: How to Live This Year as If It Were Your Last; Guided Meditations, Explorations, and Healings; A Gradual Awakening: An Introduction to Buddhist Meditation;* and *Meetings at the Edge: Dialogues with the Grieving and Dying, the Healing and the Healed.* He has the ability to speak to profound truths in a way that releases our incomplete understanding. He is a peaceful and loving person whose work reflects the compassion and wisdom he humbly offers.

When someone is dying, the patient's family is often struggling to keep them alive, which is what I did with Cindy. It seems so right to try and keep this person alive. But what would alert you that maybe this is a form of denial, that the person is dying, and that maybe you should shift to dying?

These are multileveled issues you are getting into. First of all, if you or your loved one is ill, around the time that they are no longer ambulatory, a certain level of denial drops away from us. For example, the mother may have breast cancer that's metastasized, but the kids are saying, "You look so great. You're cooking all the meals, you're still Mommy, you couldn't be too sick." That's the point at which not only is the patient's natural denial broken, but also the family's. That's the point at which you discuss exactly the question you're asking: "What if I get worse? What do you want me to do?" In our fear of death, it's understandable that we don't take the opportunity [to confront the dying process] because everyone in the house may be desirous of [keeping the person alive], but they [the family] need just another impetus, just another nanosecond of energy to get that ball rolling, and then it will. That's when hospice work or a third party may help.

If you haven't done that, if you are with your loved one, and she [or he] is dying, and you haven't really had the chance to talk over what might be wanted, that already is an indication [of denial]. For that person, their dignity was to not talk about death. People ask us very frequently, "How do I take away the denial of my loved one?" But why *would* you take away the denial of your loved one? What's going on in *you?* It may be *your* denial that's causing the problem, not theirs. It's their dignity. If your mom lived her life not wanting to talk about death, what makes you think she's going to want to talk about it on her deathbed? It's wishful thinking. We have to watch that wishful thinking, because there's also the possibility that we want them to die our death for us; we may want them to have a beautiful death, according to all the recipes.

But the problem with this stuff about conscious dying is it may create a model in people's minds, and any model is unreal. It lacks the flow of the truth. You come to the point where your friend is dying and ask, "Well, what should I do now? Should I change course?" I think, at that point, it's more important—or as important—for you to investigate your own motivation, because maybe you're not fully accepting your friend's nonacceptance.

We live in a culture that is a little late. It's not surprising that these things are asked. I think that if it happens, one of the things one can do is just sit quietly next to the bed and try to get a sense, beyond the fear, maybe get a sense, maybe listen to that person's heart. Because sometimes you may be with a loved one who cannot speak as they die, and then you are going to have to trust your connection with them.

Some of us have preconceived ideas or scenarios about many things, including dying. You call these models. Could you give an example?

I don't know if we want to get into this now, but Freud was trying to understand, using examples of models, why, in the analysis of people he was working with, the subconscious, the "underdream," if you will, has no concept for its own death. Now, he had an extraordinary piece of information in the palm of his hand, which we can call a "fact." So, he had this fact that the subconscious mind has no concept for its own death. Imagine if he had stayed in the scientific modality of "What does this mean?" But instead he had a model. He came to this investigation with a model, which is extremely unscientific.

One of the exquisite things about science—and it's part of the living spirit that's died in science, as it has in religion—is that you came to it with great "don't know": you come to it open to the truth. But Freud said, "I have a model that we die." So, if you're coming to it with a model "we die," you can't find the truth. Maybe the reason the underdream, the subconscious, has no concept for its own death [is that] we don't die. He had it. It slipped through.

How about talking briefly about some of the other schools of thought with regard to death. In Buddhism, they talk about a transitional period, right?

If a person asked, "How do I know that we exist after death?" I would say, "What difference does it make?" Because what's happening is fear in this moment. We can get into the philosophical overlays that squash emotion and keep us in the mind, keep us superficial. But I would say, "What's going on now?" I mean, this is fear of the future, but that fear exists in the present, and we work with that. So, when the future comes, it's just as [the poet] Kabir says: "What is found now, is found then. If you make love with the divine now," he says, "in the next life you'll have a face of satisfied desire," and if you do not, perhaps in the next life you'll simply have an empty apartment in the city of death. If you live in an empty apartment in the city of life, you'll probably live in an empty apartment in the city of death. If you live in the world of love and you care, as often as possible [here, in this world], that's how a good day will be there. I try only to speak from my own experience. I know, beyond a shadow of a doubt, that you survive the body. We're not the body. There are ways of experiencing in the body that you are other than the body—with the "ah"—a dying meditation, the "ah" breath.

It doesn't matter [if we exist after death]. Does it affect mercy and kindness now? If it does, something is out of balance. Here is an example: a nineteen-year-old boy [with a] brain tumor. He is the last [of his siblings] out of the house. He can just see his apartment down the street. Just got his car. Diagnosis: brain tumor. And I meet him about a year later, shaved head, scars, very thin, in a hospital, looks like it's the last round, and he is ripped, angry. He says, "What is going to happen when I die?" And I say, "I don't know." "But," he says, "it is pretty common knowledge among the hundreds of thousands of people who have had near-death experiences—a tunnel, a light, a great being... Will I be able to make thundering and lightning out?" I said, "I don't know. You may, but my sense is that the experience, the process of death itself, will bring things into order, into understanding, into acceptance, in a way that is very difficult. You may have nothing to be angry with. You may not feel that kind of separation. I don't know." He says, "What about this light?" I say, "There are people who speak of meeting a being of light, of power, of compassion, of intelligence." He says, "Oh, I'm going to meet Spock!"

Now, if I said, "No, it's Jesus," or " No, it's Buddha," you waste a person, and you might as well leave the room, because that's the end of that conversion. I think a lot of dying children see Leonardo, a Mutant Ninja Turtle, as their image. I think that's exactly how you work with someone who is dying. You would not overlay a Buddhist idea, you would not overlay a Christian idea, a Hebrew idea. You'd hear what *their* idea is of the sacred, and you go with it. And they are right, and they may be an atheist. So, their idea of the sacred could be nothing but clear, intellectual, concise thought. Well, imagine having ten to fifteen times the concentration you have now. How is that for clear, concise thought?

What do you feel are the most important things for a person to do to deal with their own death?

You mean if someone got a prognosis today—"You've got six months to live"—they could give you the answer to that question a second after they leave the doctor's office. Your priorities clarify. That is the beauty of letting go of the denial of death, because that gives an immediacy to your life. You know just what to do. Some people want to go to a monastery, some people want at last to see Grandma or their kids or their old lovers. Some may want to make amends. Some people may finish their twelve-step program. Some people may take their first step on a new program. It's so different for [different] people.

A fellow I know has a tumor in his chest, and every once in a while you'll see him touching it. "See what's happening?" he says. "This is the wish-fulfilling gem. If I want to live my life, this keeps reminding me it's all mine. I have never been so free. I have never been beyond my conditioning of my boundaries so much as I am in this moment, knowing that I have only six months to live. I have never been so alive."

How about when you're up to the point when somebody is dying—is there something that you would tell a person who is dying that he or she should do?

No. Why? Why would you tell them? If they haven't asked, it's not your problem. And you will be creating a tension in the room that increases the resistance to the moment and therefore creates suffering. If a person doesn't ask, and you see the person having a hard time, you can ask them how you can help or what's bothering them or if there's anything that would help right now. And you'd find out what's lacking. And it may be, "Oh, if my daughter was here." It may be, "Oh, if we used a different fabric softener on my pillowcases, smell them." So, at least you'll find, at a certain level, what is blocking the imagined comfort. Then, you can maybe get to other levels of, "Is there someone you want to meet?"

Now there is another level, too, perhaps: "Is there someone you don't want to see? Is there someone you don't want in this room while you're going through this very vulnerable, very personal process?" And this addresses the point of having an *ombudsman*, having a "samurai," as it were—you know, there are a lot of people dying who do not want to be with their mother or their father for all kinds of reasons. Usually it's abuse at some level. Some people don't want to be with their children, some people don't want to see their best friend or their old lovers. If you're sick and you're in bed, you just don't have the energy.

If you're sick, you've got your job cut out for you: to put your energy back into yourself and to try to touch with mercy. You're trying to break the old conditioning of sending hatred into pain, and maybe opening it to mercy. Someone else can do the social work: they can stand at the door. I've seen this quite literally, people standing at the door and saying, "I'm sorry, you cannot see your son."

"I'm going to see my son."

"I'm sorry, he really says this is what he needs."

"I'm going to call the district attorney."

"There's the phone. Could you do it quietly? You're not getting in the room."

Do you recommend hospices or dying at home, and what kind of suggestions do you have for dying at home?

Dying at home is the best. Really the best. Surveys showed that three out of four people said they would prefer to die at home. In actuality, three out of four people die in a hospital. Now, if your loved one died in a hospital, and you didn't know what alternatives were available, I don't want you to think that you've done something amiss. You did what you could. But, for most people, it's better to be at home, even children. You may think it isn't good for your other children. But, if you still are giving your other children a lot of attention, it's all right, it's really good, it is wonderful.

I know a mother of a friend of ours who was dying. This was about fifteen years ago in Long Island, when this kind of thing was not spoken of in polite company. And people walked out and they brought her home from the hospital in the last weeks of her life. She had cancer, extended abdomen, no hair. And all her friends and all the people in the neighborhood she'd lived in for a long time would cross the street when they walked by the house. That was the house of death. That was a real no-no. But, because of social convention, when they went to the house, they brought lasagna or brownies. They would always come to the door—with trepidation—and be greeted by both sons with, "Oh, come in, come in." And there was more warmth, care, and love, and less bickering in that house than they had ever seen. Then they started crossing the street to the same side as the house when they walked by because that was the house of love, not the house of death. It changed people's attitudes in the neighbor-hood, and after that many more people in that neighborhood were brought home to die.

How does one work through grief?

How do you work through grief? You feel what you feel. You know, it's amazing, that we're asked that question so much. What is more natural than grief? It just shows how far we've gotten from our true heart, that we have to ask what to do with pain. That is sadder than the fact that there is pain in the world. When you're sad, you cry; when you're happy, you laugh. You know what this country needs is temples for grieving. Maybe old-style Greek temples, open, no roof, temples where we reflect, where people just sit and weep, weep into the water. I think that the closest we've gotten to that is the AIDS quilt and the Vietnam memorials. They are spectacular examples of what this country needs.

How is grief more than just a death of a significant other? You have talked about "the pains of a lifetime" and how "every loss is recapitulated in all other previous losses."

Grief is a loss reaction. When it's someone you love, they've become a mirror for your heart. When you love someone, when they come in the room, you say, "I love you," you're just overwhelmed with this whoosh of love. Now, that's not coming from them, that's coming from you. So, when a loved one dies, you lose the mirror for your heart. You break a level of connection with yourself, with the heart. It's hard to get by the mind. Someone's heart is drawing you by the mind, and when that heart's not there, there's a terrible loss of self. When someone says, "When she died, I lost part of myself," you bet that's exactly what happened.

Freud said, "The best I can do is replace your neurotic misery with common, normal, human unhappiness." I think I'll go to a dif-ferent doctor, thank you! It's not enough. It's not enough. And, it cer-tainly isn't our potential, which is much greater than that. We can have that common, everyday, ordinary grief, that normal human unhappiness, floating in something so enormous that, for a lack of a better term, in exasperation, you'd call God. But it's just the com-monality of all beings; it's just "beingness," consciousness, *awe.* Our grief keeps us from experiencing what we have lost because what we have *really* lost, our greatest pain, is our homesickness for God. Now you might not call it "God"; you can call it your "true nature," you can call it "the comfort of the heart." Any words will do, because it's beyond language, it's prelinguistic, prebirth.

So in working with grief, [remember that] everyone has a loss. Even if a person was born in such a way, in such a place, that they had no loss, everyone around them is going to die. And I think that one of the things that's exquisite about dropping the denial of death is that then you see how much grief there is, and you really get to work. You really start to uncover what you want, the source of satisfaction.

You talk of "healing into life and death." How is dying a healing opportunity?

When we speak of healing, we're not speaking necessarily of cure; we're talking about the human heart coming to completion. We're talking, too, about the level at which the mind sinks into the heart, where there's room in our heart for our pain and for each other's pain. That's a healing. The healing we took birth for is the healing, in a sense, of the interdependence of all sentient beings. In the beginning, it's [just] a sense, but later it's a direct experience [because] it becomes so common.

One of the bizarre things about spirituality is that when you start, ooh, it's all so special, so different, so mystical. We read too deeply into it. There's really almost nothing to it. It's just "ah." It's so common, so ordinary. The most extraordinary part of us, everyone has.

In dying, too, there are the opportunities for healing. You have the willingness to finish business with forgiveness. So, you may have a lot of forgiveness in the house, a lot of psychological healing. A healing that opens past obstructions to more "don't know," to more trust in the spirit of things and one's own spirit. We use healing to approach with mercy and awareness areas that we have withdrawn from in anger and fear and judgment. Instead of ostracizing, we embrace. We start embracing our pain, opening to it, approaching it. We ask, What is it? What's its texture in the body? What shapes does it take? Where is it held, and how? What tone does it use in the mind? Every state of mind has a personality—what kind of language, what feeling, what's the stipulation in the mind? How long does it take before it repeats its game, before it comes back to the very beginning again? Because each time you see it come back to the beginning, you get a sense that it is impersonal. There is tremendous growth when you see that the shadows you understood as personal are just old flotsam, passing through. Great freedom [in realizing this]; the sign of healing is liberation. The sign of cure is only that you can take another step. I don't mean to get too flippant about this: you don't want to die; you don't want to leave your children; you don't want her to die; and you'd give up all the growth and all the evolution if she could be hanging out in this room now. But given that she isn't hanging out in this room now, and that you both will be hanging out in the same room eventually, you might as well bring into that room all the gifts possible.

You talk about love as the optimum strategy for healing, how it's a no-lose proposition.

Because love is acceptance. If you're in pain and I love you, you don't have to be different. That's wonderful if you're ill, to have someone in the room for whom you don't have to perform. You don't have to be a dying person or a healing person or a song. Just being, in that room.

What is the process of opening to the heart?

In opening to the heart, probably the first thing you're going to have to do is grief work. It's the same as with any healing—you have to do the grief work first. You have to see what obstacles exist to our natural capacity to heal. We know that grief coagulates, creates a calcified, outer layer of thought around pain, mental as well as physical. In the same way that physical pain attracts grief, grief can attract physical pain. And sometimes we get pretty sick when we are ailing. Then we get in a tight fix—where's our inner resources?

So, we're teaching people to take the medicine, feel it on their tongue, feel the water go down, feel it drop into their stomach, feel it start to build as heat and light, and then, to direct it. What we do is we get the person to focus on the tumor, so that they have a connection between consciousness and the sensations generated there. Then we use the sensations as a conduit through which to send the medicine. We see people getting well quicker, we see medication acting more directly, more powerfully, and we see fewer side effects in some people.

What approach should people take toward their illness?

I say treat your body, your sick body, as though it were your only child, and touch it with mercy. Notice how you are sending fear into the illness, naturally.

What are the characteristics of those people that seem to be "successful," best able to heal themselves?

You're asking about the characteristics of people who heal themselves. Well, the people who come to us are not the general population. Usually our people come to us for help in preparing to die. In the course of starting to approach the unfinished business around pain, mental and physical, and working with forgiveness, we have seen that certain people—often the ones who most thoroughly allow themselves to open to death—heal. Maybe the resistance around their illness fell away. Maybe in letting go of the denial to that degree, the immediacy of life was so strong in them that it overwhelmed the other imbalance. I don't see any general characteristics among them, because I've seen people who've done absolutely no work on themselves *get cured*. But I've only seen people who have been willing to work on themselves *heal*.

I have seen people get cured, and in their cure they have reinforced their aggressive qualities so much that they have driven their family away. And they're alive, and alone, and have created enormous unfinished business with their cure. I've seen other people with the same illness enter it, open to it, be merciful and kind instead of sending aggression and fear and hatred into it. Finished business. I've seen people send forgiveness into their tumors, and I've seen them get well, and they're really well, they're cured. But even more exquisite, even more stunning, is how *healed* they are.

And I've seen the opposite. I've seen people heal, heal, heal in hospitals—openings like you'd expect in a monastery—but their body continues to degenerate, and they die. So I don't understand quite what "cure" is. I know what healing has to do with—touching with mercy, opening with softness to the hard, using the heart to connect with the disheartened. That's healing.

What is your one message to give to people?

What's the meaning of life? I'll tell you the meaning of life, it's "pay attention." If you do that, everything else will become clear. Of course, even if you do that, things *won't* clear sometimes. It's hard enough when you *are* trying to keep your heart open, to be present. There's so much debris, so much momentum, so much unfinished business in the mind and the body.

But if you're not trying, you don't have a chance. If you're waiting for it to happen spontaneously, yes, it may. But you won't be able to do anything with it. You won't be able to integrate that experience, because you won't have the capacity to be grounded in other realms, in other states of consciousness. If you're doing spiritual work and not psychological work, the insights that arise are difficult to integrate into yourself, much less into the world. It's hard to bring them into the service of other sentient beings because there are so many obstacles in the mind to clarity. If you do only spiritual work and you say, "Ahh, the psychological is just *mind*, that's not *me*, and since mind is not self I won't bother with it," then, you have a strong spiritual practice, but not much psychological opening. In that case, when you have profound insight, you can't integrate it. It just keeps bouncing. And the mind may actually cause you to lose your ground, instead of [your] being more grounded—of sending roots down through your psychology into your body, heart, mind.

Conversely, if you're doing only psychological work and not spiritual work, that psychological work will tend to lead you to think that you're the mind and the body, and, therefore, you won't draw on other levels of your being—the levels out of which the satisfaction you're searching for psychologically can be attained. So it's both. It's not either psychology or spirit, it's whole. And it's more difficult to be a whole human being than to be a saint. Most of the saints are pretty neurotic, pretty one-sided. It is better just to teach our children to listen and observe.

[All interviews have been edited for length and clarity.]

Information regarding Stephen Levine's books, tapes and workshops is available through

Warm Rock Tapes
P.O. Box 108
Chamisal, NM 87521
Phone: 800-731-HEAL (800-731-4325)

Conclusion

Action Steps for Your Healing Journey

The sheer volume of information, choices, and emotions that face cancer patients can be overwhelming. To help keep things organized, the following is a summary of key issues. It includes recommendations for action and study, and treatment information to be considered.

You should add to the list any issues, concerns, and action items that are especially pertinent to your situation.

Commit to life

Consider these questions: Are you committed to living? Are there internal barriers to healing? Are you willing to do what it takes to heal from cancer?

Get support

Take care of yourself. Don't go it alone. Find people to share with—family, friends, cancer help lines. Get involved with a support group. Shop for a group you are comfortable with. They vary widely in quality. Find one that shares your treatment philosophy.

Do your homework

Read, ask questions. Research, gather information. Use a research service (see Recommended Reading and References).

Find the doctor who is right for you

Find a doctor you are comfortable with and who shares your treatment philosophy. You will have easier access to more treatment options if your doctor agrees to help you with testing should you choose to go an alternative or complementary route.

Be assertive with doctors and hospitals regarding your needs

Remember that doctors and hospitals are your paid consultants; they work for you (even though many do not act this way). You have a right to know, to have your questions answered, and to be treated with respect. When you visit the doctor's office or hospital, consider bringing someone along for support, to help you get what you need.

Get a second opinion, know your exact diagnosis, your five-year survival odds, and your tumor aggressiveness

Always get a second opinion regarding your diagnosis and treatment options. Find out your exact diagnosis, your five-year survival odds, and the aggressiveness of your tumor. This information gives you an idea of how much time you have and the odds of surviving your cancer with conventional treatment alone.

Participate in a residential program or workshop

Residential programs and cancer workshops, if you can find one that fits your budget and needs, can provide tremendous amounts of information and support for cancer patients (see Resources, section D).

Avoid complacency

Do not be lulled into a false sense of security if your cancer is in remission or if your survival odds are good. The cancer may or may not return. If you have had cancer, you are obviously prone to it and susceptible to its return. The fact that it has occurred at all is a warning. You want to do everything you can to keep cancer from returning, because when it returns and spreads is when it is most often deadly. Learn what you can do now to keep it from returning later.

Time your breast cancer surgery if you are premenopausal

Time your surgery to take advantage of potential increased survival odds (see "Timing of Breast Cancer Surgery for Premenopausal Women," chapter 3).

Minimize the effects of chemotherapy and radiation

Do what you can to minimize the damage and side effects of chemotherapy and radiation and to rebuild your immune system. Your immune system is what's going to help keep you alive in the long haul. The goal is to keep cancer from returning.

Consider pretesting chemotherapies

Have your doctor acquire a large enough biopsy to allow for chemosensitivity testing to see which chemotherapy will work best on your cancer.

Time the delivery of chemotherapy

The time of day a chemotherapeutic drug is given has an impact on the effectiveness of the drug and on how much damage is caused to the immune system and other cells in the body. Optimal times for delivery of many common chemotherapies are known (see "Circadian Timing of Chemotherapy Delivery," chapter 3). Ask your doctor for, or find a hospital capable or willing to set you up with, a programmable drug infusion pump for your chemotherapy.

Find out about clinical trials

There is a new group of very promising gene and immunotherapies, including vaccines and biologics, being tested in clinical trials. Your doctor should be aware of any new appropriate treatments or clinical trials for your type of cancer. You can also call 1-800-4-CANCER. Be sure to ask for the survival statistics and information on side effects for these individual therapies so you can evaluate them properly.

Consider alternatives

If you have a cancer that is untreatable with conventional therapy, and your odds for survival are basically nil, then what have you got to lose by trying an alternative? Your money? You won't need it if you don't survive, and most alternatives are actually less expensive than conventional treatments, although not covered by insurance. If you have the cash, consult with a research service about alternatives. They have a better idea of which ones work for specific cancers. If possible, pretest alternatives (see "Pretesting Therapeutic Agents for Your Specific Cancer," chapter 3). Talk to those who have used the treatment—in person, by phone, or on the Internet.

Be sure you have access to testing

Have a reliable test done, prior to beginning a course of alternative treatment, to establish a baseline for your cancer. Then have another test done after you have been on the treatment to see if the alternative is working or if you need to change course.

Use complementary therapies

Look into what supplemental treatments are available to complement your primary treatment, whether it is some herbal supplement for your immune system, or psychological counseling. Like Dr. Lawrence LeShan says, a few extra votes can make all the difference in a close election.

Find an experienced psychotherapist

One of the most important and overlooked supplemental treatments is psychotherapy. Many hospitals offer counseling to cancer patients, and although this is useful for coping with many aspects of cancer and some quality-of-life issues, it will seldom, if ever, replace what a seasoned therapist can do. Emotional issues can have a profound impact on our immune system and our ability to heal. Find a therapist skilled in finding out "what's right with you"—what gifts you have to give to the world—and begin living the life you want. At the very least, you will increase the quality and satisfaction of your life, and at best you may save it.

Live Life and Love Yourself

Take the time to live life fully. Don't put off the activities that bring you deep satisfaction. If you have to, schedule time just for what you want to do. Remember to love yourself, treat yourself gently and with kindness. Take time to appreciate the things you like about yourself and your life. If you believe in a Higher Power, take comfort in the knowledge that you are eternally loved and cared for.

Resources

Section A
Comprehensive Cancer Centers

Alabama

University of Alabama at Birmingham Comprehensive Cancer Center
1824 Sixth Avenue South, Room 237
Birmingham, AL 35294-3300
Phone: 205-934-5077

Arizona

University of Arizona Cancer Center
1501 North Campbell Avenue
Tucson, AZ 85724
Phone: 520-626-7925

California

Jonsson Comprehensive Cancer Center
UCLA
Factor Building, Room 8-684
10833 Le Conte Avenue
Los Angeles, CA 90095
Phone: 310-825-5268

USC/Norris Comprehensive Cancer Center
University of Southern California
1441 East Lake Avenue, Room 815, MS #83
Los Angeles, CA 90033
Phone: 323-865-0816

UCI Cancer Center
University of California at Irvine
101 The City Drive
Building 23, Rt. 81, Room 406
Orange, CA 92868
Phone: 714-456-6310

Colorado

University of Colorado Cancer Center
University of Colorado Health Science Center
4200 East 9th Avenue, Box B188
Denver, CO 80262
Phone: 303-315-3007

Connecticut

Yale University Comprehensive Cancer Center
333 Cedar Street, Box 208028
New Haven, CT 06520
Phone: 203-785-4371

District of Columbia

Lombardi Cancer Research Center
Georgetown University Medical Center
3800 Reservoir Road, NW
Washington, DC 20007
Phone: 202-687-2110

Illinois

Robert H. Lurie Cancer Center
Northwestern University
303 East Chicago Avenue
Olson Pavilion 8250
Chicago, IL 60611
Phone: 312-908-5250

Maryland

The Johns Hopkins Oncology Center
600 North Wolfe Street, Room 157
Baltimore, MD 21287
Phone: 410-955-8822

Massachusetts

Dana-Farber Cancer Institute
44 Binney Street, Room 1628
Boston, MA 02115
Phone: 617-632-2155

Michigan

University of Michigan Comprehensive Cancer Center
1500 East Medical Center Drive
Ann Arbor, MI 48109
Phone: 313-936-1831

Barbara Ann Karmanos Cancer Institute
Executive Office
4100 John R. Street
Detroit, MI 48201
Phone: 313-993-7777

New Hampshire

Norris Cotton Cancer Center
Dartmouth-Hitchcock Medical Center
One Medical Center Drive, Hinman Box 7920
Lebanon, NH 03756-0001
Phone: 603-650-6300

New York

Cancer Research Center
Albert Einstein College of Medicine
Chanin Building, Room 209
1300 Morris Park Avenue
Bronx, NY 10461
Phone: 718-430-2302

Roswell Park Cancer Institute
Elm and Carlton Streets
Buffalo, NY 14263
Phone: 716-845-2389

Kaplan Cancer Center
New York University Medical Center
550 First Avenue

New York, NY 10016
Phone: 212-263-6485

Memorial Sloan-Kettering Cancer Center
1275 York Avenue
New York, NY 10021
Phone: 212-639-6561

Herbert Irving Comprehensive Cancer Center
College of Physicians and Surgeons
Columbia University
177 Fort Washington Avenue
6th Floor, Room 435
New York, NY 10032
Phone: 212-305-8602

North Carolina

Duke Comprehensive Cancer Center
Duke University Medical Center
P.O. Box 3843
Durham, NC 27710
Phone: 919-684-5613

UNC Lineberger Comprehensive Cancer Center
University of North Carolina School of Medicine, CB-7295
102 West Drive
Chapel Hill, NC 27599-7295
Phone: 919-966-3036

Cancer Center
Wake Forest University
Bowman Gray School of Medicine
Medical Center Boulevard
Winston-Salem, NC 27157
Phone: 336-716-7971

Ohio

Case Western Reserve University
University Hospitals Ireland Cancer Center
11100 Euclid Avenue
Cleveland, OH 44106
Phone: 216-844-8562

Comprehensive Cancer Center
Arthur G. James Cancer Hospital
Ohio State University
A445 Staring Loving Hall
320 West 10th Avenue
Columbus, OH 43210
Phone: 614-293-7518

Pennsylvania

Fox Chase Cancer Center
7701 Burholme Avenue
Philadelphia, PA 19111
Phone: 215-728-2781

University of Pennsylvania Cancer Center
16th Floor Penn Tower
3400 Spruce Street
Philadelphia, PA 19104
Phone: 215-662-6065

University of Pittsburgh Cancer Institute
3471 Fifth Avenue, Suite 201
Pittsburgh, PA 15213
Phone: 412-692-4670

Texas

The University of Texas
M. D. Anderson Cancer Center
1515 Holcombe Boulevard, Box 91
Houston, TX 77030
Phone: 713-792-6000

San Antonio Cancer Institute
8122 Datapoint Drive, Suite 250
San Antonio, TX 78229
Phone: 210-616-5590

Vermont

Vermont Regional Cancer Center
University of Vermont
1 South Prospect Street

Burlington, VT 05401
Phone: 802-656-4414

Washington

Fred Hutchinson Cancer Research Center
1100 Fairview Avenue, North
P.O. Box 19024, LY301
Seattle, WA 98109-1024
Phone: 206-667-4305

Wisconsin

University of Wisconsin
Comprehensive Cancer Center
600 Highland Avenue, Room K4/610
Madison, WI 53792
Phone: 608-263-8610

Section B

Support Groups

Many hospitals now offer cancer support groups. They vary greatly in quality. Review your experience of the support you are receiving, and do not hesitate to leave if you feel that the group is not beneficial for you.

National Coalition for Cancer Survivorship (NCCS)
1010 Wayne Avenue
Fifth Floor
Silver Spring, MD 20910
Phone: 301-650-8868

Provides support for persons wishing to locate or form self-help groups; assists survivors with insurance and employment problems; provides a variety of excellent free publications (some in Spanish), including booklets on working with your health care team, insurance, and The National Networking Directory of Cancer Support Services.

The American Self-Help Clearinghouse
Northwest Covenant Medical Center
25 Pocono Road
Denville, NJ 07834
Phone: 973-625-9565

The American Self-Help Clearinghouse is a national organization that can refer you to national self-help groups, as well as to state and regional clearinghouses that have information on local groups that are not members of national networks.

The Wellness Community (National Office)
2716 Ocean Park Blvd., Suite 1040
Santa Monica, CA 90405
Phone: 310-314-2555

The Wellness Community is an excellent national network of cancer support centers. These centers offer informal sharing groups, ongoing weekly groups facilitated by psychotherapists, family groups, relaxation and visualization sessions, workshops and lectures, exercise and nutrition classes, and groups designed to facilitate the exchange of information in specialized areas of concern to cancer patients.

American Cancer Society
1599 Clifton Road, N.E.
Atlanta, GA 30329
Phone: 1-800-ACS-2345

The American Cancer Society conducts and supports programs of research, education, and service to cancer patients. Public education activities include publication of a variety of pamphlets and educational programs. Look in your phone book for the chapter nearest you to determine services available locally.

Anderson Network
M. D. Anderson Cancer Center
1515 Holcombe Boulevard, Box 216
Houston, TX 77030
Phone: 1-800-345-6324

The Anderson Network offers hope, resources, and understanding to those facing cancer. Through a free telephone service called Network Telephone Lines, it links cancer patients with others who have survived.

R. A. Bloch Cancer Foundation Hot Line
4410 Main Street
Kansas City, MO 64111
Phone: 800-433-0464

Supplies referrals to hospitals that provide multidisciplinary second opinions and support organizations and provides free copies of Richard Bloch's books, *Fighting Cancer; Cancer, There's Hope;* and *Guide for Cancer Supporters* (all excellent).

Cancer Care, Inc.
1180 Avenue of the Americas
New York, NY 10036
Phone: 212-221-3300

National Cancer Counseling Line
Phone: 800-813-HOPE

Offers professional social work, counseling, and guidance to help patients and families cope with the emotional and psychological consequences of cancer.

Cancer Hope Network
2 North Road, Suite A
Chester, NJ 07930
Phone: 1-877-HOPENET

Offers personal, one-to-one emotional support to cancer patients (and their families) who are undergoing chemotherapy and/or radiation treatment, from trained and certified volunteers who have survived the treatment themselves.

Support for Specific Cancers

Breast Cancer

Y-Me
212 West Van Buren
Chicago, IL 60607
Phone: 800-221-2141

Y-Me provides information, hot-line counseling, educational programs, and self-help meetings for breast cancer patients, their families, and friends. Available by calling their toll-free, twenty-four-hour hot line. Upon request, trained volunteers, all whom have had breast cancer, are matched to callers with similar backgrounds and experiences. Y-Me is conservative on unconventional cancer treatment issues. Chapters vary greatly in the quality of the service they provide.

Y-Me Men's Support Line
Men with family or friends with breast cancer who need support can call the Y-Me hot line and request to speak to a male counselor. The counselor most closely matched in experience to the caller will return the call within twenty-four hours.

Save Ourselves
P.O. Box 1100
Sacramento, CA 95812
Phone: 800-422-9747

Provides referral for newly diagnosed cancer patients and their loved ones to breast cancer services and consultants.

Oral, Head, and Neck Cancer

Support for People with Oral and Head and Neck Cancer, Inc. (SPOHNC)
P.O. Box 53
Locust Valley, NY 11560-0053
Phone: 516-759-5333
Website: www.spohnc.org
Email: info@spohnc.org

Self-help programs of support. Addresses the broad emotional, psychological, and humanistic needs of these cancer survivors, empowering each to take an active role in his or her recovery.

Prostate Cancer

US TOO International, Inc.
930 North York Road, Suite 50
Hinsdale, IL 60521-2993
Phone: 708-323-1002 or 800-808-7866

Provides prostate cancer survivors and their families emotional and educational support through an international network of chapters.

Patients Advocates for Advanced Cancer Treatments (PAACT)
1143 Parmelee, NW
Grand Rapids, MI 49504
Phone: 616-453-1477

Association for both patients and physicians for diagnostic and therapeutic treatment of prostate cancer.

Note: There may be other cancer-specific support organizations. To find a support organization for your cancer, contact organizations like the National Coalition for Cancer Survivorship or The American Self-Help Clearinghouse.

Section C
Cancer Organizations

National Cancer Institute (NCI) Office of Cancer Information and Cancer Education
31 Center Drive MSC2580
Building 31, Room 10A16
9000 Rockville Pike
Bethesda, MD 20982-2580
Phone: 800-4-CANCER (800-422-6237)
Cancer Fax Line: 301-402-5874
(For help with Cancer Fax, call 301-496-7600.)

Provides a nationwide telephone service for cancer patients and their families and friends, the public, and health care professionals. Answers questions, sends booklets about cancer, and provides Physician Data Query printouts. Cancer Fax provides treatment guidelines, with current data on prognosis, relevant staging and histologic classifications, and news and announcements for important cancer-related issues. Call Cancer Fax from a fax machine.

Organizations Dedicated to Specific Cancers

American Brain Tumor Association
2720 River Road, Suite 146
Des Plaines, IL 60018
Phone: 800-886-2282

Offers free services, including publications about brain tumors, support group lists, referral information, and a pen pal program.

American Lung Association
1740 Broadway
New York, NY 10019-4374
Phone: 212-315-8700

Dedicated to conquering lung disease and promoting lung health.
National Brain Tumor Foundation
785 Market Street, Suite 1600
San Francisco, CA 94103
Phone: 800-934-CURE

Pursues goals of providing support and education for brain tumor patients and finding a cure through research.

United Ostomy Association, Inc.
19772 Macarthur Boulevard, Suite 200
Irvine, CA 92612
Phone: 714-660-8624 or 800-826-0826

Association of ostomy chapters dedicated to complete rehabilitation.

National Kidney Cancer Association
1234 Sherman Avenue, Suite 203
Evanston, IL 60202
Phone: 847-332-1051

Works to increase the survival of kidney cancer patients and improve their care by providing information, sponsoring research, and acting as an advocate on behalf of patients.

International Myeloma Foundation
2129 Stanley Hills Drive
Los Angeles, CA 90046
Phone: 800-452-CURE

Promotes education for physicians and patients about myeloma and its treatment and management. Funds research, holds clinical and scientific conferences, and publishes a quarterly newsletter, *Myeloma Today*.

Leukemia Society of America
600 Third Avenue
New York, NY 10016
Phone: 800-955-4LSA (educational materials)
Phone: 212-573-8484 (general information)

Dedicated to seeking the cause and eventual cure of leukemia and related cancers. Nationwide programs include research, patient aid, and public and professional education. Offers local family-support-group programs free of charge, open to patients, families, families, and friends.

Lymphoma Research Foundation of America, Inc.
8800 Venice Boulevard, Suite 207
Los Angeles, CA 90034
Phone: 310-204-7040

A research organizations that also provides a support system for lymphoma patients across the country.

Patient Advocates for Advanced Cancer Treatments
P.O. Box 1656
Grand Rapids, MI 49501
Phone: 616-391-2534

Provides an intelligent review of the latest developments in prostate cancer treatment. Will send a comprehensive packet of information on prostate cancer to anyone who requests it.

The Skin Cancer Foundation
245 Fifth Avenue, Suite 1403
New York, NY 10016
Phone: 212-725-5176

Provides public and medical education programs and support for medical training and research. Helps reduce incidence and mortality of skin cancer.

National Alliance of Breast Cancer Organizations (NABCO)
9 East 37th Street, 10th Floor
New York, New York 10016
Phone: 212-889-0606

Source of information on breast cancer. Advocates for legislative and regulatory concerns of breast cancer community.

Miscellaneous Cancer Organizations

Corporate Angel Network
Westchester County Airport
1 Loop Road
White Plains, NY 10604
Phone: 914-328-1313

Nationwide service that transports cancer patients and a family member or friend free of charge to or from a "recognized cancer treatment," using empty seats on corporate aircraft. The only requirements of the service are that the patient be able to walk unassisted and that no life support or other special services be required.

Bone Marrow Transplant Newsletter
1985 Spruce Avenue
Highland Park, IL 60035
Phone: 847-831-1913
Fax: 847-831-1943
Website: www.bmtnews.org
Email: help@bmtnews.org

Publishes bimonthly newsletter and a book on issues of concern to
patients. Provides attorney referrals for those having difficulty obtaining
reimbursement for their treatment.

National Marrow Donor Program
3433 Broadway Street, N.E., Suite 400
Minneapolis, MN 55413
Phone: 800-MARROW-2

A congressionally authorized network that maintains a computerized data
bank of available tissue-typed marrow donors nationwide.

Bone Marrow Transplant Family Support Network
P.O. Box 845
Avon, CT 06001
Phone: 800-826-9376

Enables families to feel connected when coping with a transplant decision,
daily routines prior to and following transplants, and follow-up care after a
transplant.

National Bone Marrow Transplant Link (BMT Link)
29209 Northwestern Highway, #642
Southfield, MI 48034
Phone: 800-LINK-BMT

Reduces the burdens of those affected by bone marrow transplantation
and promotes public understanding and peer support.

Note: Some information regarding Support and Cancer Organizations has
been provided by *Coping Magazine,* a quarterly magazine of cancer issues
and support:

Coping Magazine
P.O. Box 682268
Franklin, TN 37068-2268
Phone: 615-790-2400

Section D
Cancer Programs

The following are organizations that offer cancer-related trainings, seminars, and residential programs for cancer support, evaluation of treatment options, relaxation or pain management training, and exploration of psychological aspects of cancer:

Beth Israel Deaconess Medical Center
Division of Behavioral Medicine
110 Francis Street, Suite 1A
Boston, MA 02215
Phone: 617-632-9530
Fax: 617-632-7383

Outpatient clinic designed to help patients deal with the stress of the disease and of the side effects of treatment, and to help the patient take an active role in care. Teaches relaxation response meditation and use of "creative imagination."

U. Mass. Memorial Health Care
Stress Reduction Clinic/Center for Mindfulness
Shaw Building
55 Lake Avenue, North
Worcester, MA 01655
Phone: 508-856-2656
Fax: 508-856-1977

Eight-week-long course that teaches people with a wide range of medical diagnoses how to deal with chronic stress, pain, and illnesses. Program is training in mindfulness mediation.

Wellspring Center for Life Enhancement
173 Mt. Auburn Street
Watertown, MA 02472
Phone: 617-924-8515
Fax: 781-862-0555

Provides variety of services, including support groups, consultations to discuss choices, and training in relaxation and visualization.

Optimum Health Institute
6970 Central Avenue
Lemon Grove, CA 92045
Phone: 619-464-3346

Offers a three-week course in "rejuvenation" through diet, various health practices, and attitudinal adjustment.

Vega Study Center
1511 Robinson Street
Oroville, CA 95965
Phone: 530-533-4777

Offers a twelve-day "Cancer and Healing" program every other month. Program centers on macrobiotic diet but also covers psychosocial aspects, communication, and home remedies.

Bristol Cancer Help Centre
Grove House
Clifton, Bristol BS8 4PG
England
United Kingdom
Phone: 011-44-117-974-3216

Offers a week-long residential course that uses group support, meditation, visualization, and self-help techniques to assist patients in adjusting to the experience of cancer and cancer treatment. Scholarships are available.

The Yarra Valley Living Centre
P.O. Box 77G
Yarra Junction
Victoria 3797, Australia
Phone: 011-61-3-5967-1730

The ten-day program focuses on developing self-help techniques and coping skills. Included are techniques for: transforming fear into positive action; developing peace of mind; managing personal pain; improving communication skills; and committing to personal development through disease. A workshop uses drawing to gain personal insight. A five-day follow-up program focuses on problem solving and application of the techniques.

Commonweal Cancer Help Program
P.O. Box 316
Bolinas, CA 94924
Phone: 415-868-0970
Website: www.commonwealhealth.org

One-week retreat for people seeking physical, mental, emotional, and spiritual healing in the face of cancer. Participants are given the opportunity to reduce the fear and stress associated with cancer, to examine personal beliefs and behaviors that do not contribute to well-being, and to explore choices in treatment that may be beneficial. Some scholarships are available.

Simonton Cancer Center: New Patient Program
P.O. Box 890
Pacific Palisades, CA 90272
Phone: 310-459-4434

A five-day educational and psychotherapeutic session for cancer patients and their spouses conducted by O. Carl Simonton and staff of therapists. Simonton pioneered mental imagery as an complementary approach to cancer.

Section E
Websites

Information on Conventional Treatment

American Cancer Society
  www.cancer.org

Oncolink: University of Pennsylvania Cancer Center
  cancer.med.upenn.edu/

Cancerweb
  www.graylab.ac.uk/cancerweb.html

Guide to Internet Resources for Cancer
  www.ncl.ac.uk/~nchwww/guides/clinks1.htm

Medicine On-Line
  www.meds.com/index.html

Cancer Link
  www.personal.u-net.com/~njh/cancer.html

Cancer Sites of General Interest
  www.cancernews.com/sites.html

Information on Both Conventional and Alternative/Complementary Treatments

Cancer Guide: Steven Dunn's Cancer Information Page
  cancerguide.org/

Commonweal
  www.commonwealhealth.org

Cancer Patient Resources
  www.charm.net/~kkdk/

Nonprofit Resources Catalog: Cancer
  www.clark.net/pub/pwalker/Health_and_Human_Services/Cancer/

CANCER: Increasing Your Odds for Survival
  www.cancersurvival.com

Information on Alternative/Complementary Treatments

Office of Alternative Medicine (OAM)
   altmed.od.nih.gov/oam/about/

OAM Center for Alternative Medicine Research in Cancer
   www.sph.uth.tmc.edu/utcam

Center for Empirical Medicine
   home.earthlink.net/~emptherapies/index.html

Moss Reports
   www.ralphmoss.com/

Alternative Medicine
   alternativemedicine.com

People Against Cancer
   peopleagainstcancer.com

Cancer Support Groups

National Coalition for Cancer Survivorship Home Page
   www.cansearch.org

American Self-Help Clearinghouse Source Book Online
   www.cmhc.com/selfhelp/

Cancer Survivors Online
   www.ahamade.com/CancerSurvivors/

Cancer Care
   www.cancercareinc.org/

A Cancer Survivor's Story: Live the Pain, Learn the Hope
   www.dmgi.com/treelife.html

Cancer Research Resources

National Cancer Institute: CancerNet (MEDLINE @ PDQ)
   cancernet.nci.nih.gov/Arc Information on Cancer
   www.arc.com/cancernet/cancernet.html

National Coalition of Cancer Survivorship: Can Search
   www.cansearch.org/cansearch/canserch.htm

Highline Community Hospital Health Care Network
   http://www.hchnet.org/

Recommended Reading
and References

Recommended Reading

Many good books on cancer have been included as resources for the various topics in this resource guide. The following are a few of the best books I highly recommend.

For information on dealing with understanding cancer, dealing with the diagnosis, doctors, insurance, conventional treatment, and other issues facing cancer patients and their families:

Marion Morra and Eve Potts, *Choices: Realistic Alternatives in Cancer Treatment* (New York: Avon Books, 1980).

National Coalition for Cancer Survivorship, *A Cancer Survivor's Almanac: Charting Your Journey,* Ed. Barbara Hoffman, J.D. (Minneapolis, MN: Chronimed Publishing, 1996).

For information on combining conventional and complementary treatment approaches:

Michael Lerner, Ph.D., *Choices in Healing: Integrating the Best of Conventional and Complementary Approaches to Cancer* (Cambridge, MA: MIT Press, 1994). This book can be viewed in its entirety on the Internet at: www.commonwealhealth.org.

For those looking into alternative and complementary approaches:

John Fink, *Third Opinion: An International Directory to Alternative Therapy Centers for the Treatment of Cancer and Other Degenerative Diseases* (Garden City Park, NY: Avery Publishing Group, 1997).

Ralph W. Moss, Ph.D., *Cancer Therapy: The Independent Consumer's Guide to Nontoxic Treatment and Prevention* (New York: Equinox Press, 1992).

267

W. John Diamond, M.D., and W. Lee Cowden, M.D., with Burton Goldberg, *An Alternative Medicine Definitive Guide to Cancer* (Tiburon, CA: Future Medicine Publishing, 1997).

For those interested in psychological aspects of cancer:

Lawrence LeShan, Ph.D., *Cancer as a Turning Point: A Handbook for People with Cancer, Their Families, and Health Professionals* (New York: Dutton/ Penguin, 1989).

For those interested in the psychological and spiritual aspects of healing:

Joan Borysenko, Ph.D., *Guilt Is the Teacher, Love Is the Lesson* (New York: Warner Books, 1990).

Stephen Levine, *Healing into Life and Death* (New York: Anchor/Doubleday, 1987).

For those dealing with the end of life:

Stephen Levine, *Who Dies? An Investigation of Conscious Living and Conscious Dying* (New York: Anchor/Doubleday, 1982).

References

Part 1   Diagnosis and Empowerment

Chapter 1   Understanding Cancer

American Cancer Society. *Cancer Facts and Figures—1998.* Atlanta, GA: American Cancer Society, 1998. Booklet.

Breast Cancer: Patients' Survival. Washington, DC: GAO, 1989. Publication PEMD-89-9.

Buckman, Robert, M.D. *What You Really Need to Know About Cancer: A Comprehensive Guide for Patients and Their Families.* Baltimore, MD: Johns Hopkins University Press, 1995.

Cancer Patient Survival: What Progress Has Been Made? Washington, DC: GAO, 1987. Publication PEMD-87-13.

Cancer Treatment: National Cancer Institute's Role in Encouraging the Use of Breakthroughs. Washington, DC: GAO, 1988. Publication PEMD-89-4BR.

Cancer Treatment 1975–85: The Use of Breakthrough Treatments for Seven Types of Cancer. Washington, DC: GAO, 1988. Publication PEMD-88-12BR.

Gordon, James S., M.D. *Manifesto for a New Medicine: Your Guide to Healing Partnerships and the Wise Use of Alternative Therapies.* Reading, MA: Perseus Press, 1996.

Marchetti, Albert, M.D. *Beating the Odds: Alternative Treatments That Have Worked Miracles Against Cancer.* Chicago, IL: Contemporary Books, 1988.

McKhann, Charles F., M.D. *The Facts About Cancer: A Guide for Patients, Family, and Friends.* Englewood Cliffs, NJ: Prentice-Hall, 1981.

Morra, Marion, and Eve Potts. *Choices: Realistic Alternatives in Cancer Treatment.* New York: Avon Books, 1980.

National Cancer Institute with National Institutes of Health. *SEER Cancer Statistics Review, 1973–1992: Tables and Graphs.* Bethesda, MD: National Cancer Institute, 1990. NIH Booklet 96-2789.

National Institutes of Health. *Cancer: Rates and Risks.* 4th ed. Bethesda, MD: NIH, 1996.

———. *Fact Book: National Cancer Institute.* Bethesda, MD: NIH, 1998. NIH Booklet 98-512.

Chapter 2 Dealing with Cancer

American Cancer Society. *Listen with Your Heart: Talking with the Cancer Patient.* Atlanta, GA: American Cancer Society, 1996. Booklet.

Benjamin, Harold H., Ph.D. *The Wellness Community Guide to Fighting for Recovery from Cancer.* New York: Putnam, 1987.

Bloch, Richard A. *Cancer... There's Hope.* Kansas City, MO: R. A. Bloch Cancer Foundation, 1981.

Bloch, Richard A., and Annette Bloch. *Fighting Cancer: A Step-by-Step Guide to Helping Yourself Fight Cancer.* Kansas City, MO: R. A. Bloch Cancer Foundation, 1985.

Bracken, Jeanne Munn. *Children with Cancer: A Comprehensive Guide for Parents.* New York: Oxford University Press, 1986.

Cancer Treatments Your Insurance Should Cover. Rockville, MD: Association of Community Cancer Centers, 1995. Booklet.

Ferguson, Tom, and Edward J. Madara. *Health Online: How to Find Health Information, Support Groups, and Self-Help Communities in Cyberspace.* Reading, MA: Perseus Press, 1996.

Fink, John. *Third Opinion: An International Directory to Alternative Therapy Centers for the Treatment of Cancer and Other Degenerative Diseases.* Garden City Park, NY: Avery Publishing Group, 1997.

Fiore, Neil, Ph.D. *The Road Back to Health: Coping with the Emotional Aspects of Cancer.* Rev. ed. Berkeley, CA: Celestial Arts, 1990.

Kauffman, Danette G. *Surviving Cancer.* Washington, DC: Acropolis Books, 1989.

LeShan, Lawrence, Ph.D. *Cancer as a Turning Point: A Handbook for People with Cancer, Their Families, and Health Professionals.* New York: Dutton/Penguin, 1989.

Matthews-Simonton, Stephanie. *The Healing Family: The Simonton Approach for Families Facing Illness.* New York: Bantam, 1984.

Morra, Marion, and Eve Potts. *Choices: Realistic Alternatives in Cancer Treatment.* New York: Avon Books, 1980.

———. *The Prostate Cancer Answer Book: An Unbiased Guide to Treatment Choices.* New York: Avon Books, 1996.

———. *Triumph: Getting Back to Normal When You Have Cancer.* New York: Avon Books, 1990.

Nader, Ralph, William M. Shernoff, and Ruth Chew. *How to Make Insurance Companies Pay Your Claims, and What to Do If They Don't.* Mamaroneck, NY: Hastings House Publishers, 1990.

National Cancer Institute. *Facing Forward: A Guide for Cancer Survivors.* Bethesda, MD: National Cancer Institute, 1990. NIH Booklet 90-2424.

———. *Taking Time: Support for People with Cancer and the People Who Care About Them.* Bethesda, MD: National Cancer Institute, 1990. NIH Booklet 92-2059.

———. *Understanding the Immune System.* Bethesda, MD: National Cancer Institute, 1990. NIH Booklet 90-529.

———. *When Someone in Your Family Has Cancer.* Bethesda, MD: National Cancer Institute, 1992. NIH Booklet 92-2685.

National Coalition for Cancer Survivorship. *A Cancer Survivor's Almanac: Charting Your Journey.* Ed. Barbara Hoffman, J.D. Minneapolis, MN: Chronimed Publishing, 1996.

———. *Teamwork: The Cancers Patient's Guide to Talking with Your Doctor.* Silver Spring, MD: National Coalition for Cancer Survivorship, 1991. Brochure.

———. *What Cancer Survivors Need to Know About Health Insurance.* Minneapolis, MN: Chronimed Publishing, 1993.

Pollner, Fran. "Part of the Primary Cancer Mix: Cancer Patients." *Medical World News* (October 1990).

Schine, Gary L., with Ellen Berlinsky, Ph.D. *Cancer Cure: The Complete Guide to Finding and Getting the Best Care There Is.* New York: Kensington Books, 1993.

Siegel, Bernie S., M.D. *Love, Medicine, & Miracles: Lessons Learned About Self-Healing from a Surgeon's Experience with Exceptional Patients.* New York: Harper & Row, 1986.

Viatical Settlements: A Guide for People with Terminal Illnesses. Free from FTC Public Reference Branch, 6th Street and Pennsylvania Avenue, NW, Room 130, Washington, DC 20580.

What You Need to Know About Accelerated Benefits. Free from the National Insurance Consumer Hot Line at 800-942-4242.

Part 2   Treatment

Chapter 3   Conventional Treatments

Abrams, Martin B., et al. "Early Detection and Monitoring of Cancer with the Anti-Malignin Antibody Test." *Cancer Detection and Prevention* 18, no. 1 (1994): 65–78.

Austin, Steve, N.D., and Cathy Hitchcock, M.S.W. *Breast Cancer: What You Should Know (But May Not Be Told) About Prevention, Diagnosis, and Treatments.* Rocklin, CA: Prima Publishing, 1994.

Badwe, R. A., et al. "Timing of Surgery During Menstrual Cycle and Survival of Premenopausal Women with Operable Breast Cancer." *Lancet* 337 (May 25, 1991): 1261–64.

Cramer, Andrew B., M.D., and Eugene A. Woltering, M.D. "Chemosensitivity Testing: A Critical Review." *Critical Reviews in Clinical Laboratory Studies* 28 (1991): 405–12.

DeVita, Vincent T., Jr., M.D., Samuel Hellman, M.D., and Steven A. Rosenberg, M.D., Ph.D., eds. *Cancer: Principles and Practice of Oncology.* Philadelphia: Lippincott, 1992. See article on pp. 2666–86, "The Application of Circadian Chronobiology to Cancer Treatment."

Diamond, W. John, M.D., and W. Lee Cowden, M.D., with Burton Goldberg. *An Alternative Medicine Definitive Guide to Cancer.* Tiburon, CA: Future Medicine Publishing, 1997.

Evans, Richard A., M.D. *Making the Right Choice in Cancer Surgery: Treatment Options in Cancer Surgery.* Garden City Park, NY: Avery Publishing Group, 1995.

Fink, John. *Third Opinion: An International Directory to Alternative Therapy Centers for the Treatment of Cancer and Other Degenerative Diseases.* Garden City Park, NY: Avery Publishing Group, 1997.

Finkel, Maurice, M.S., Ed.D. *Fresh Hope in Cancer: Natural Methods for Prevention, Treatment, and Control of Cancer.* N. Devon, England: Health Science Press, 1998.

Folkman, Judah. "Fighting Cancer by Attacking Its Blood Supply." *Scientific American* 275, no. 3 (Sept. 1996): 150–54.

Folkman, J., T. Boehm, T. Browder, and M.S. O'Reilly. "Anti-angiogenic Therapy of Experimental Cancer Does Not Induce Acquired Drug Resistance." *Nature* 390 (Nov. 27, 1997): 404–407.

Fulder, Stephen. *How to Survive Medical Treatment: A Holistic Guide to Avoiding the Risks and Side Effects of Conventional Medicine.* Woodstock, NY: Beekman Publishers, 1995.

Hagen, Andreas A., M.D., et al. "Menstrual Timing of Breast Cancer Surgery." *American Journal of Surgery* 104 (Mar. 1998): 245–61.

Harpham, Wendy Schlessel, M.D. *Diagnosis: Cancer: Your Guide Through the First Few Months.* New York: Norton Books, 1998.

Hellman, Samuel, and Everett E. Vokes. "Advancing Current Treatments for Cancer." *Scientific American* 275, no. 3 (Sept. 1996): 118–23.

Hrushesky, William J. M., M.D. "Breast Cancer, Timing of Surgery, and the Menstrual Cycle: Call for Prospective Trial." *Journal of Women's Health* 5, no. 6 (Nov. 6, 1996): 555–66.

———. "Circadian Cancer Therapy." *Journal of Clinical Oncology* 11 (July 1995): 1403–17.

———. "Circadian Timing of Cancer Chemotherapy." *Science* 228 (Apr. 1985): 73–75.

Hrushesky, William J. M., M.D., et al. "Chronotherapy of Cancer: A Major Drug-Delivery Challenge." *Advanced Drug Delivery Reviews* 9 (1992): 1–83.

Hrushesky, William J. M., M.D., et al. "Menstrual Influence on Surgical Cure of Breast Cancer." *Lancet* 2 (Oct. 21, 1989): 949–52.

Hrushesky, William J. M., M.D., ed. *Circadian Cancer Therapy.* Boca Raton, FL: CRC Press, 1994.

Leone, L. A., M.D., et al. "Predictive Value of the Fluorescent Cytoprint Assay (FCA): A Retrospective Correlation Study of In Vitro Chemosensitivity and Individual Responses to Chemotherapy." *Cancer Investigation* 9, no. 5 (1991): 491–503.

Levi, Francis, et al. "Randomised Multicentre Trial of Chronotherapy with Oxaliplatin, Fluorouracil, and Folinic Acid in Metastatic Colorectal Cancer." *Lancet* 350 (Sept. 6, 1997): 681–86.

Love, Susan M., M.D., with Karen Lindsey. *Dr. Susan Love's Breast Book.* 2d ed. Reading, MA: Addison-Wesley, 1995.

McGinn, Kerry A., R.N., N.P., and Pamela J. Haylock, R.N. *Women's Cancers: How to Prevent Them, How to Treat Them, How to Beat Them.* 2d ed. Alameda, CA: Hunter House, 1998.

Meitner, Patricia A., Ph.D. "The Fluorescent Cytoprint Assay: A New Approach to In Vitro Chemosensitivity Testing." *Oncology* 5, no. 9 (Sept. 1991): 75–88.

Morra, Marion, and Eve Potts. *Choices: Realistic Alternatives in Cancer Treatment.* New York: Avon Books, 1980.

Moss, Ralph W., Ph.D. *The Cancer Industry: The Classic Exposé on the Cancer Establishment.* New York: Equinox Press, 1996.

———. *Cancer Therapy: The Independent Consumer's Guide to Nontoxic Treatment and Prevention.* New York: Equinox Press, 1992.

National Cancer Institute. *Chemotherapy and You: A Guide to Self-Help During the Treatment.* Bethesda, MD: National Cancer Institute, 1993. Publication 94-1136.

————. *Eating Hints: Recipes and Tips for Better Nutrition During Cancer Treatment.* Bethesda, MD: National Cancer Institute, 1992. Publication 92-2079.

————. *Radiation Therapy and You: A Guide to Self-Help During the Treatment.* Bethesda, MD: National Cancer Institute, 1990. Publication 91-2227.

————. *Understanding the Immune System.* Bethesda, MD: National Cancer Institute, 1990. Publication 90-529.

————. *What Are Clinical Trials All About?* Bethesda, MD: National Cancer Institute, 1992. Publication 92-2709.

National Coalition for Cancer Survivorship. *A Cancer Survivor's Almanac: Charting Your Journey.* Ed. Barbara Hoffman, J.D. Minneapolis, MN: Chronimed Publishing, 1996.

National Institutes of Health. *Fact Book: National Cancer Institute.* Bethesda, MD: NIH, 1998. NIH Booklet 98-512.

Old, Lloyd J. "Immunotherapy for Cancer." *Scientific American* 275, no. 3 (Sept. 1996): 136–43.

Oliff, Allen, Jackson B. Gibbs, and Frank McCormick. "New Molecular Targets for Cancer Therapy." *Scientific American* 275, no. 3 (Sept. 1996): 144–49.

Rosenberg, Steven A., M.D., Ph.D. *The Transformed Cell: Unlocking the Mysteries of Cancer.* New York: Avon Books, 1992.

Schine, Gary L., with Ellen Berlinsky, Ph.D. *Cancer Cure: The Complete Guide to Finding and Getting the Best Care There Is.* New York: Kensington Books, 1993.

Senie, Ruby T., Ph.D., et al. "Timing of Breast Cancer Excision During the Menstrual Cycle Influences Duration of Disease-free Survival." *Annals of Internal Medicine* 115, no. 5 (Sept. 1991): 337–403.

Taneja, Samir, et al. "Immunotherapy for Renal Cell Carcinoma: The Era of Interleukin-2–Based Treatment." *Urology* 45 (June 1995): 911–23.

Ulrich, Abel, M.D. *Chemotherapy of Advanced Epithelial Cancer: A Critical Survey.* Stuttgart: Hippokrates Verlag, 1990.

Chapter 4   Alternative Treatments

Becker, Robert, M.D. *Cross Currents: The Promise of Electromedicine, The Perils of Electropollution.* Los Angeles, CA: J. P. Tarcher, 1990.

Bird, Christopher. *The Galileo of the Microscope: The Life and Trials of Gaston Naessens.* St. Lambert, Quebec: Les Presses de l'Université de la Personne, 1990.

Clark, Hulda Regehr, P.L.D., N.P. *The Cure for All Cancers: With 100 Case Histories*. San Diego, CA: New Century Press, 1993.

Does Cartilage Cure Cancer? The Shark and Bovine Cartilage Controversy: An Independent Assessment. Working paper by Vivekan Don Flint and Michael Lerner. Available from Michael Lerner's Commonweal program and at their website: www.commonwealhealth.org.

Diamond, W. John, M.D., and W. Lee Cowden, M.D., with Burton Goldberg. *An Alternative Medicine Definitive Guide to Cancer*. Tiburon, CA: Future Medicine Publishing, 1997.

Elias, Thomas D. *The Burzynski Breakthrough: The Century's Most Promising Cancer Treatment . . . and the Government's Campaign to Squelch It*. Los Angeles, CA: General Publishing Group, 1997.

Ferguson, Tom, and Edward J. Madara. *Health Online: How to Find Health Information, Support Groups, and Self-Help Communities in Cyberspace*. Reading, MA: Perseus Press, 1996.

Fink, John. *Third Opinion: An International Directory to Alternative Therapy Centers for the Treatment of Cancer and Other Degenerative Diseases*. Garden City Park, NY: Avery Publishing Group, 1997.

Glassman, Judith. *The Cancer Survivors and How They Did It*. New York: Dial Press, 1983.

Lane, William, Ph.D., and Linda Comac. *Sharks Don't Get Cancer*. Garden City Park, NY: Avery Publishing Group, 1992.

———. *Sharks Still Don't Get Cancer*. Garden City Park, NY: Avery Publishing Group, 1996.

Lerner, Michael, Ph.D. *Choices in Healing: Integrating the Best of Conventional and Complementary Approaches to Cancer*. Cambridge, MA: MIT Press, 1994.

Moss, Ralph W., Ph.D. *Cancer Therapy: The Independent Consumer's Guide to Nontoxic Treatment and Prevention*. New York: Equinox Press, 1992.

Naiman, Ingrid. *Cancer Salve and Suppositories: A Botanical Approach to Treatment*. Santa Fe, NM: Seventh Ray Press, 1997.

National Institutes of Health. *Alternative Medicine: Expanding Medical Horizons*. Washington, DC: Government Printing Office, 1994. Publication 94-066.

Nordenstrom, Bjorn, M.D. "Electrochemical Treatment of Cancer, I: Variable Response to Anodic and Cathodic Fields." *American Journal of Clinical Oncology* 12 (1989): 530–36.

———. "Electrochemical Treatment of Cancer, II: Effect of Electrophoretic Influence on Adriamycin." *American Journal of Oncology* 13 (1990): 75–88.

Office of Alternative Medicine. *Alternative Medicine: Expanding Medical Horizons.* Washington, DC: Government Printing Office, 1994. Stock no. 017-040-00537-7.

Office of Technology Assessment. *Unconventional Cancer Treatments.* Washington, DC: Government Printing Office, 1990. Report OTA-H-405.

Pelton, Ross, Ph.D., and Lee Overholser, Ph.D. *Alternatives in Cancer Therapy: The Complete Guide to Nontraditional Treatments.* New York: Simon & Schuster, 1994.

Prudden, John, M.D. "The Treatment of Human Cancer with Agents Prepared from Bovine Cartilage." *Journal of Biological Response Modifiers* 4 (Dec. 1985): 551–84.

Taubes, Gary. "An Electrifying Possibility." *Discover* (Apr. 1986).

Trull, Louise. *The CanCell Controversy: Why Is a Possible Cure for Cancer Being Suppressed?* Norfolk, VA: Hampton Roads, 1993.

Walters, Richard. *Options: The Alternative Cancer Therapy Book.* Garden City Park, NY: Avery Publishing Group, 1993.

Young, Alan. *The Cancer Puzzle: An In-Depth Explanation of Cancer and Its Prevention, Treatment, and Causes.* Portland, OR: Frank Amato Publications, 1994.

Zakarian, Beverly. *The Activist Cancer Patient: How to Take Charge of Your Treatment.* New York: John Wiley & Sons, 1996.

Zhang, Dai-zhao. *Treatment of Cancer by Integrated Chinese-Western Medicine.* Boulder, CO: Blue Poppy Press, 1989.

Chapter 5   Complementary and Supplemental Treatments

Altman, Nathaniel. *Oxygen Healing Therapies for Optimum Health and Vitality.* Rochester, VT: Healing Arts Press, 1995.

Balch, James F., M.D., and Phyllis A. Balch, C.N.C. *Prescription for Nutritional Healing: A Practical A–Z Reference.* Garden City Park, NY: Avery Publishing Group, 1997.

Baten, Abdul, et al. "Inositol-Phosphate-Induced Enhancement of Natural Killer Cell Activity Correlates with Tumor Suppression." *Carcinogenesis* 10 (1989): 1595–98.

Begin, Michael E., et al. "Differential Killing of Human Carcinoma Cells Supplemented with n-3 and n-6 Polyunsaturated Fatty Acids." *Journal of the National Cancer Institute* 77 (1986): 1053–62.

Begin, Michael E., et al. "Polysaturated Fatty Acid–Induced Cytotoxicity Against Tumor Cells and Its Relationship to Lipid Peroxidation." *Journal of the National Cancer Institute* 80, no. 3 (1988).

Berry, Linda. *Internal Cleansing: Rid Your Body of Toxins and Return to Vibrant Health.* Rocklin, CA: Prima Publishing, 1997.

Boik, J. *Cancer and Natural Medicine: A Textbook of Basic Science and Clinical Research.* Princeton, MN: Oregon Medical Press, 1995. See pp. 117–20, 160.

Budwig, Johanna, Ph.D. *Flax Oil as a True Aid Against Arthritis, Heart Infarction, Cancer, and Other Diseases.* Vancouver, BC: Apple Publishing, 1996.

———. *The Oil Protein Diet Cookbook: Use of Oils in Cooking.* Vancouver, BC: Apple Publishing, 1996.

Cameron, Ewan, and Linus Pauling. *Cancer and Vitamin C.* Rev. ed. Philadelphia, PA: Camino Books, 1993.

Charnow, Jody A. "New Evidence That Green Tea Helps Fight Cancer." *Medical Tribune News Service* (Apr. 16, 1997).

Chein, Edmund, et al. "Acupuncture and Cancer." *American Journal of Acupuncture* 4 (1976).

The Chlorella Source Book. A binder full of research articles, available for a small fee. Health and Happiness Publishing, Phone: 800-694-2224.

Colbin, Annemarie. *Food & Healing.* Rev. ed. New York: Ballantine Books, 1996.

Diamond, W. John, M.D., and W. Lee Cowden, M.D., with Burton Goldberg. *An Alternative Medicine Definitive Guide to Cancer.* Tiburon, CA: Future Medicine Publishing, 1997.

Dreizen, S., et al. "Nutritional Deficiencies in Patients Receiving Cancer Chemotherapy." *Postgraduate Medicine* 161 (1987): 163–68.

Eisenberg, David, M.D., and Thomas Lee Wright. *Encounters with Qi: Exploring Chinese Medicine.* New York: Norton, 1995.

Eisenberg, David, M.D., et al. "Unconventional Medicine in the United States." *New England Journal of Medicine* 328 (Jan. 28, 1993): 246–51.

Enstrom, James E., et al. "Vitamin C Intake and Mortality Among a Sample of the United States Population." *Epidemiology* 3, no. 3 (1994): 194–202.

Fink, John. *Third Opinion: An International Directory to Alternative Therapy Centers for the Treatment of Cancer and Other Degenerative Diseases.* Garden City Park, NY: Avery Publishing Group, 1997.

Finkel, Maurice, M.S., Ed.D. *Fresh Hope in Cancer: Natural Methods for Prevention, Treatment, and Control of Cancer.* N. Devon, England: Health Science Press, 1978.

Fujiki, H., et al. "New Antitumor Promoters: (-)-Epigallocatechin Gallate and Sarcophytols A and B." *Basic Life Sciences* (1990): 205–12.

Fulder, Stephen. *How to Survive Medical Treatment: A Holistic Guide to Avoiding the Risks and Side Effects of Conventional Medicine.* Woodstock, NY: Beekman Publishers, 1995.

Gazella, Karolyn. *Buyer—Be Wise!: The Consumer's Guide to Buying Quality Nutritional Supplements.* Green Bay, WI: IMPAKT Communications, 1998.

Gold, J. "Hydrazine Sulfate: A Current Perspective." *Nutritional Cancer* 9 (1987): 59–66.

———. "Use of Hydrazine Sulfate in Terminal and Preterminal Cancer Patients: Results of Investigational New Drug (Ind) Study in 84 Evaluable Patients." *Oncology* (1975): 1–10.

Haas, Robert, M.S. *Permanent Remissions: Life-Extending Diet Strategies That Can Help Prevent and Reverse Cancer, Heart Disease, Diabetes, and Osteoporosis.* New York: Pocket Books, 1997.

Herbal Remedies for Cancer. Working paper by Vivekan Don Flint and Michael Lerner. Available from Michael Lerner's Commonweal program and at their website: www.commonwealhealth.org.

Hoffer, A., M.D., et al. "Hardin Jones Biostatistical Analysis of Mortality Data for Cohorts of Cancer Patients with a Large Fraction Surviving at the Terminal of the Study and a Comparison of Survival Times of Cancer Patients Receiving Large Regular Oral Doses of Vitamin C and Other Nutrients with Similar Patients Not Receiving Those Doses." *Journal of Orthomolecular Medicine* 5, no. 3 (1990): 143–54.

Hoffer, Abram, M.D., and Linus Pauling. *Vitamin C and Cancer.* Kingston, Ontario: Quarry Press, forthcoming 1998.

Hsu, Hong-Yen. *Treating Cancer with Chinese Herbs.* New Canaan, CT: Keats Publishing, 1993.

Hunsberger, Eydie Mae, with Chris Loeffter. *How I Conquered Cancer Naturally.* Garden City Park, NY: Avery Publishing Group, 1992.

Jochems, Ruth, and Linus Pauling. *Dr. Moerman's Anti-Cancer Diet: Holland's Revolutionary Nutritional Program for Combating Cancer.* Garden City Park, NY: Avery Publishing Group, 1990.

Keane, Maureen B., and Daniella Chace. *What to Eat If You Have Cancer: A Guide to Adding Nutritional Therapy to Your Treatment Plan.* Chicago, IL: Contemporary Books, 1996.

Kennedy, Ann. "The Evidence for Soybean Products as Cancer Preventive Agents." *Journal of Nutrition* 125 (1995): 733–43.

Kobayashi, H., et al. "Antimetastatic Effects of PSK, A Protein-Bound Polysaccharide Obtained from Basidiomycetes: An Overview." *Cancer Epidemiology, Biomarkers & Prevention* 4, no. 3 (1995): 275–81.

Kushi, Michio, with Edward Esko. *The Macrobiotic Approach to Cancer: Towards Preventing Cancer with Diet and Lifestyle.* Garden City Park, NY: Avery Publishing Group, 1991.

———. *The Macrobiotic Cancer-Prevention Cookbook.* Wayne, NJ: Avery Publishing Group, 1988.

Lad, Usha, and Vasant Lad. *Ayurvedic Cooking for Self-Healing.* 2d ed. Albuquerque, NM: Ayurvedic Press, 1997.

Lamm, Donald, et al. "Megadose Vitamins in Bladder Cancer: A Double-Blind Clinical Trial." *Journal of Urology* 151 (Jan. 1994): 21–26.

Laux, Marcus, M.D. *Power Over Cancer: The 1996 Handout.* Potomac, MD: Phillips Publishing, 1996.

Lerner, Michael, Ph.D. *Choices in Healing: Integrating the Best of Conventional and Complementary Approaches to Cancer.* Cambridge, MA: MIT Press, 1994.

Lockwood, M. K., et al. "Apparent Partial Remission of Breast Cancer in 'High Risk' Patients Supplemented with Nutritional Antioxidants, Essential Fatty Acids, and Coenzyme Q10." *Molecular Aspects of Medicine* 15, suppl. (1995): 231–40.

Lopez, D. A., M.D., R. Michael Williams, M.D., Ph.D, and K. Miehlke, M.D. *Enzymes: The Foundation of Life.* Charleston, SC: The Neville Press, 1994.

McCabe, Ed. *Oxygen Therapies: A New Way of Approaching Disease.* Morrisvillle, NY: Energy Publications, 1988.

Merchant, Randall, et al. "Dietary Chlorella Pyrenoidosa for Patients with Malignant Glioma: Effects on Immunocompetence, Quality of Life, and Survival." *Phytotherapy Research* 4 (1990): 220–30.

Moss, Ralph W., Ph.D. *Cancer Therapy: The Independent Consumer's Guide to Nontoxic Treatment and Prevention.* New York: Equinox Press, 1992.

Nash, Barbara. *From Acupressure to Zen: An Encyclopedia of Natural Therapies.* Alameda, CA: Hunter House, 1996.

National Institutes of Health. *Alternative Medicine: Expanding Medical Horizons.* Washington, DC: Government Printing Office, 1994. Publication 94-066.

Office of Alternative Medicine. *Alternative Medicine: Expanding Medical Horizons*. Washington, DC: Government Printing Office, 1994. Stock no. 017-040-00537-7.

Office of Technology Assessment. *Unconventional Cancer Treatments*. Washington, DC: Government Printing Office, 1990. Report OTA-H-405.

Pauling, Linus. *How to Live Longer and Feel Better.* New York: Avon Books, 1986.

Pelton, Ross, Ph.D., and Lee Overholser, Ph.D. *Alternatives in Cancer Therapy: The Complete Guide to Nontraditional Treatments.* New York: Simon & Schuster, 1994.

Quillin, Patrick, and Noreen Quillin. *Beating Cancer with Nutrition: Clinically Proven and Easy-to-Follow Strategies to Dramatically Improve Your Quality and Quantity of Life and Increase Chances for a Complete Remission.* New York: Nutrition Times Press, 1998.

Shamsuddin, A., M.D. "Comparison of Pure Inositol Hexaphosphate and High Bran Diet in the Prevention of DMBA-Induced Rat Mammary Carcinogenesis." *Nutrition and Cancer* 28 (1997): 7–13.

Shamsuddin, A., M.D., et al. "Minireview IP-6: A Novel Anti-Cancer Agent." *Live Science* 61 (1987): 343–54.

Thompson, Trula, M.D., M.Ph. "Re-Engineering the RDAs: Do the RDAs Support Surviving or Thriving?" *Adjuvant Nutrition in Cancer Treatment Symposium* (Sept. 28–30, 1995).

Torisu, M., et al. "Significant Prolongation for Disease-Free Period Gained by Oral Polysaccharide K (PSK) Administration After Curative Surgical Operation of Colorectal Cancer." *Cancer Immunology and Immunotherapy* 31 (1990): 261–68.

Toufexis, Anastasia. "The New Scoop on Vitamins." *Time* (Apr. 6, 1992), 54–59.

Walters, Richard. *Options: The Alternative Cancer Therapy Book.* Garden City Park, NY: Avery Publishing Group, 1993.

Wu, Z. L., et al. "Antitransforming Activity of Chlorophyllin Against Selected Carcinogens and Complex Mixtures." *Teratogenesis, Carcinogenesis, and Mutagenesis* 14 (1994): 75–81.

Yang, Jwing-Ming. *Qigong for Health and Martial Arts: Exercises and Meditation.* Jamaica Plain, MA: Yang's Martial Arts Association Publication Center, 1998.

Zhang, Dai-zhao. *Treatment of Cancer by Integrated Chinese-Western Medicine.* Boulder, CO: Blue Poppy Press, 1989.

Part 3   Mind-Body Interventions

Chapter 6   Mind-Body Therapies

Achterberg, Jeanne, Ph.D. *Imagery in Healing: Shamanism and Modern Medicine*. Boston, MA: Shambhala Publications, 1985.

Ader, Robert, David L. Felton, and Nicolas Cohen, eds. *Psychoneuroimmunology*. 2d ed. San Diego, CA: Academic Press, 1991.

Borysenko, Joan, Ph.D. *Fire in the Soul: A New Psychology of Spiritual Optimism*. New York: Warner Books, 1993.

———. *Guilt Is the Teacher, Love Is the Lesson*. New York: Warner Books, 1990.

———. *Minding the Body, Mending the Mind*. New York: Bantam Books, 1987.

Borysenko, Joan, Ph.D., and Miroslav Borysenko. *The Power of the Mind to Heal*. Carson, CA: Hay House, 1994.

Borysenko, Joan, Ph.D., and Joan Drescher. *On Wings of Light: Meditations for Awakening to the Source*. New York, Warner, 1992.

Bricklin, Mark, Mark Golin, Deborah Grandinetti, and Alexis Lieberman, eds. *Positive Living and Health: The Complete Guide to Brain/Body Healing and Mental Empowerment*. Emmaus, PA: Rodale, 1990.

Bridge, Linda, et al. "Relaxation and Imagery for Breast Cancer Patients." *British Medical Journal* 6, no. 2(Nov. 5, 1988): 28–30.

Cousins, Norman. *Anatomy of an Illness as Perceived by the Patient*. New York: Bantam, 1981.

———. *Head First: The Biology of Hope and the Healing Power of the Human Spirit*. New York: Penguin, 1990.

Dossey, Larry, M.D. *Recovering the Soul: A Scientific and Spiritual Search*. New York: Bantam, 1989.

Fiore, Neil, Ph.D. *The Road Back to Health: Coping with the Emotional Aspects of Cancer*. Rev. ed. Berkeley, CA: Celestial Arts, 1990.

Ghanta, Vithal K., et al. "Neural and Environmental Influences on Neoplasia and Conditioning of NK Activity." *Journal of Immunology* 135 (1985): 848–52.

Goleman, Daniel, Ph.D., and Joel Gurin, eds. *Mind and Body Medicine: How to Use Your Mind for Better Health*. Yonkers, NY: Consumer Reports Books, 1993.

Hay, Louise. *You Can Heal Your Life*. Santa Monica, CA: Hay House, 1984.

Hopper-Epstein, Alice, Ph.D. *Mind, Fantasy, and Healing: One Woman's Journey from Conflict and Illness to Wholeness and Health*. New York: Delacorte Press, 1989.

Jaffe, Dennis T., Ph.D. *Healing from Within.* New York: Alfred A. Knopf, 1980.

Kiecolt-Glaser, Janice, et al. "Psychosocial Modifiers of Immunocompetence in Medical Students." *Psychosomatic Medicine* 16 (Jan.–Feb. 1984): 7–14.

Korn, Errol R., and Karen Johnson. *Visualization: The Uses of Imagery in the Health Professions.* Homewood, IL: Dow Jones-Irwin, 1983.

Lane, Deforia, Ph.D., MT-B. *Music as Medicine: Deforia Lane's Life of Music, Healing and Faith.* Grand Rapids, MI: Zondervan, 1995.

Lerner, Michael, Ph.D. *Choices in Healing: Integrating the Best of Conventional and Complementary Approaches to Cancer.* Cambridge, MA: MIT Press, 1994.

LeShan, Lawrence, Ph.D. *How to Meditate: A Guide to Self-Discovery.* New York: Bantam Books, 1984.

Letter to the Editor. "Psychosocial Variables and the Course of Cancer." *New England Journal of Medicine* 313 (1985): 1354–59.

Levine, Stephen. *A Gradual Awakening: An Introduction to Buddhist Meditation.* Garden City, NY: Anchor/Doubleday, 1979.

———. *Guided Meditations, Explorations, and Healings.* New York: Anchor/Doubleday, 1991.

———. *Healing into Life and Death.* New York: Anchor/Doubleday, 1987.

Levy, S. M., Ph.D., et al. "Correlation of Stress Factors with Sustained Depression of Natural Killer Cell Activity with Predicted Prognosis in Patients with Breast Cancer." *Journal of Clinical Oncology* 5, no. 3 (1987): 349–53.

Levy, Sandra M., Ph.D., et al. "Immunological and Psychosocial Predictors of Disease Recurrence in Patients with Early-Stage Breast Cancer." *Behavioral Medicine* (Summer 1991): 67–75.

Levy, Sandra M., Ph.D., et al. "Survival Hazards Analysis in First Recurrent Breast Cancer Patients: Seven-Year Follow-Up." *Psychosomatic Medicine* 50 (1988): 520–28.

Locke, Steven E., M.D. *Psychological and Behavioral Treatments for Disorders Associated with the Immune System: An Annotated Bibliography.* New York: Institute for the Advancement of Health, 1986.

Locke, Steven E., M.D., and Douglas Colligan. *The Healer Within: The New Medicine of Mind and Body.* New York: New American Library, 1986.

Locke, Steven E., M.D., et al. *Mind and Immunity: Behavioral Immunology, an Annotated Bibliography 1976–1982.* New York: Institute for the Advancement of Health, 1983.

Locke, Steven E., M.D., et al., eds. *Foundations of Psychoneuroimmunology.* New York: Aldine, 1985.

Nhat Hanh, Thich. *Being Peace.* Berkeley, CA: Parallax Press, 1987.

Parkhill, Stephen C. *Answer Cancer: Miraculous Healings Explained: The Healing of a Nation.* Deerfield Beach, FL: Health Communications, 1995.

Plotnikoff, N. P., et al., eds. *Stress and Immunity.* Boca Raton, FL: CRC Press, 1991.

Rossi, Ernest. *The Psychobiology of Mind/Body Healing: New Concepts of Therapeutic Hypnosis.* Rev. ed. New York: W. W. Norton, 1993.

Rossman, Martin, M.D. *Healing Yourself: A Step-by-Step Program for Better Health Through Imagery.* New York: Walker, 1987.

Saltman, Joyce, Ph.D., Ed.D. *Sing a Celebration.* Watertown, MA: Ivory Tower, 1988.

Siegel, Bernie S., M.D. *Peace, Love, & Healing: Bodymind Communication and the Path to Self-Healing: An Exploration.* New York: Harper & Row, 1989.

Simonton, O. Carl, M.D., and Reid Henson, with Brenda Hampton. *The Healing Journey: The Simonton Center Program for Achieving Physical, Mental, and Spiritual Health.* New York: Bantam Books, 1992.

Simonton, O. Carl, M.D., Stephanie Matthews-Simonton, and James L. Creighton. *Getting Well Again: A Step-by-Step, Self-Help Guide to Overcoming Cancer for Patients and Their Families.* Los Angeles, CA: J. P. Tarcher, 1978.

Stapp, Will. "The Case for Imagery in Modern Medicine." *New Realities* (Mar.–Apr. 1989).

Weil, Andrew, M.D. *8 Weeks to Optimum Health.* New York: Fawcett, 1998.

Yogananda, Paramahansa. *Scientific Healing Affirmations.* Los Angeles, CA: Self-Realization Fellowship, 1998.

Zelman, Stuart, M.D., and David Bognar. *Human Operators Manual: How Feelings Work: A Psychological Primer.* Hartford, CT: n.p., 1991.

Chapter 7   Psychological Aspects of Cancer

Borysenko, Joan, Ph.D. *Minding the Body, Mending the Mind.* New York: Bantam Books, 1987.

Borysenko, Joan, Ph.D., and Miroslav Borysenko. *The Power of the Mind to Heal.* Carson, CA: Hay House, 1994.

Cassileth, Barnie, et al. "Psychosocial Correlates of Survival in Advanced Malignant Disease." *New England Journal of Medicine* 312 (June 13, 1985): 1551–55.

Cousins, Norman. *Anatomy of an Illness as Perceived by the Patient.* New York: Bantam, 1981.

———. *Head First: The Biology of Hope and the Healing Power of the Human Spirit.* New York: Penguin, 1990.

Evans, Richard I. *Jung on Elementary Psychology.* New York: Dutton, 1976.

Fiore, Neil, Ph.D. "Fighting Cancer—One Patient's Perspective." *New England Journal of Medicine* 300 (Feb. 8, 1979): 284–89.

———. *The Road Back to Health: Coping with the Emotional Aspects of Cancer.* Rev. ed. Berkeley, CA: Celestial Arts, 1990.

Goldberg, Jane G. *Deceits of the Mind and Their Effects on the Body.* New Brunswick, NJ: Transaction Publishers, 1991.

Greer, S., and T. Morris. "Psychological Attributes of Women Who Develop Breast Cancer: A Controlled Study." *Journal of Psychosomatic Research* 19 (1975): 147–53.

Greer, S., et al. "Mental Attitudes to Cancer: An Additional Prognostic Factor." *Lancet* 1 (1985): 750.

Greer, S., et al. "Psychological Response to Breast Cancer and Fifteen-Year Outcome." *Lancet* 1 (1990): 49–50.

Greer, S., et al. "Psychological Response to Breast Cancer: Effect on Outcome." *Lancet* 2 (Oct. 13, 1979): 785–87.

Holland, Jimmie C., and Julia H. Rowland. (eds.) *Handbook of Psychooncology.* New York: Oxford University Press, 1989.

Hopper-Epstein, Alice, Ph.D. *Mind, Fantasy, and Healing: One Woman's Journey from Conflict and Illness to Wholeness and Health.* New York: Delacorte Press, 1989.

LeShan, Lawrence, Ph.D. *Alternate Realities: The Search for the Full Human Being.* New York: M. Evans, 1976.

———. *Cancer as a Turning Point: A Handbook for People with Cancer, Their Families, and Health Professionals.* New York: Dutton/Penguin, 1989.

———. *How to Meditate: A Guide to Self-Discovery.* New York: Bantam Books, 1984.

———. *The Mechanic and the Gardener: How to Use the Holistic Revolution in Medicine.* New York: Holt, Rinehart & Winston, 1982.

———. *The Medium, The Mystic, and the Physicist: Toward a General Theory of the Paranormal.* New York: Penguin, 1995.

———. *The Science of the Paranormal: The Next Frontier.* Wellingborough, Northants, U.K.: Aquarian Press, 1987.

———. *You Can Fight for Your Life: Emotional Factors in the Causation of Cancer.* New York: M. Evans, 1980.

LeShan, Lawrence, Ph.D., with Henry Margenau. *Einstein's Space and Van Gogh's Sky: Physical Reality and Beyond.* New York: Macmillan, 1983.

Locke, Steven E., M.D., and Douglas Colligan. *The Healer Within: The New Medicine of Mind and Body.* New York: New American Library, 1986.

Lowen, Alexander, M.D. *The Betrayal of the Body.* London: Collier Books, 1967.

———. *Bioenergetics.* New York: Penguin, 1975.

Nash, Barbara. *From Acupressure to Zen: An Encyclopedia of Natural Therapies.* Alameda, CA: Hunter House, 1996.

Orr, Leonard, and Sondra Ray. *Rebirthing in the New Age.* Berkeley, CA: Celestial Arts, 1983.

Pelletier, Kenneth R. *Mind as Healer, Mind as Slayer: A Holistic Approach to Preventing Stress Disorders.* New York: Delacorte Press, 1977.

"Researchers Find That Optimism Helps the Body's Defense System." *New York Times* (Apr. 20, 1989).

Siegel, Bernie S., M.D. *Love, Medicine, & Miracles: Lessons Learned About Self-Healing from a Surgeon's Experience with Exceptional Patients.* New York: Harper & Row, 1986.

———. *Peace, Love, & Healing: Bodymind Communication and the Path to Self-Healing: An Exploration.* New York: Harper & Row, 1989.

Simonton, O. Carl, M.D., and Reid Henson, with Brenda Hampton. *The Healing Journey: The Simonton Center Program for Achieving Physical, Mental, and Spiritual Health.* New York: Bantam Books, 1992.

Simonton, O. Carl, M.D., Stephanie Matthews-Simonton, and James L. Creighton. *Getting Well Again: A Step-by-Step, Self-Help Guide to Overcoming Cancer for Patients and Their Families.* Los Angeles, CA: J. P. Tarcher, 1978.

Spiegal, David, et al. "Effect of Psychosocial Treatment on Survival of Patients with Metastatic Breast Cancer." *Lancet* 2 (October 14, 1989): 888–91.

Temoshok, Lydia, Ph.D., and Henry Dreher. *The Type C Connection: The Behavioral Links to Cancer and Your Health.* New York: Random House, 1992.

Zelman, Stuart, M.D., and David Bognar. *Human Operators Manual: How Feelings Work: A Psychological Primer.* Hartford, CT: n.p., 1991.

Part 4   Spirituality and Mortality

Chapter 8   Cancer and Spirituality

Baynes, Wilhelm. *The I Ching or Book of Changes.* Princeton, NJ: Princeton University Press, 1950.

Borysenko, Joan, Ph.D. *Fire in the Soul: A New Psychology of Spiritual Optimism.* New York: Warner Books, 1993.

———. *Guilt Is the Teacher, Love Is the Lesson.* New York: Warner Books, 1990.

Brennan, Barbara Ann. *Hands of Light: A Guide to Healing Through the Human Energy Field.* New York: Bantam, 1987.

———. *Light Emerging: The Journey of Personal Healing.* New York: Bantam, 1993.

Byrd, Randolph. "Positive Therapeutic Effects of Intercessory Prayer in a Coronary Care Unit Population." *Southern Medical Journal* 81, no. 7 (1988): 826–29.

Carlson, Richard, Ph.D., and Benjamin Shield, eds. *Healers on Healing.* Los Angeles, CA: J. P. Tarcher, 1989.

Chopra, Deepak, M.D. *Quantum Healing: Exploring the Frontiers of Mind/Body Medicine.* New York: Bantam, 1989.

A Course in Miracles: Combined Volume. 2d ed. Glen Ellen, CA: Foundation for Inner Peace, 1992.

Crookes, William, Sir. *Researches in the Phenomena of Spiritualism.* Litchfield, CT: Pantheon Press, 1971.

Dossey, Larry, M.D. *Be Careful What You Pray For... You Just Might Get It.* San Francisco, CA: HarperSanFrancisco, 1997.

———. *Healing Words: The Power of Prayer and the Practice of Medicine.* San Francisco, CA: HarperSanFrancisco, 1993.

———. *Prayer Is Good Medicine: How to Reap the Healing Benefits of Prayer.* San Francisco, CA: HarperSanFrancisco, 1996.

———. *Recovering the Soul: A Scientific and Spiritual Search.* New York: Bantam, 1989.

Edwards, Harry. *A Guide to the Understanding and Practice of Spiritual Healing.* Burrows Lea, England: Healer Publishing, 1974.

Edwards, Henry James. *The Healing Intelligence.* New York: Taplinger, 1971.

Jampolsky, Gerald, M.D. *Love Is Letting Go of Fear.* Berkeley, CA: Celestial Arts, 1979.

Krieger, Dolores, Ph.D., R.N. *The Therapeutic Touch: How to Use Your Hands to Help to Heal.* New York: Simon & Schuster, 1992.

Lash, John. *The Seeker's Handbook: The Complete Guide to Spiritual Pathfinding.* New York: Harmony Books, 1990.

Levine, Stephen. *Guided Meditations, Explorations, and Healings.* New York: Anchor/Doubleday, 1991.

———. *Healing into Life and Death.* New York: Anchor/Doubleday, 1987.

———. *Meetings at the Edge: Dialogues with the Grieving and Dying, the Healing and the Healed.* Garden City, NY: Anchor/Doubleday, 1984.

———. *Who Dies? An Investigation of Conscious Living and Conscious Dying.* New York: Anchor/Doubleday, 1982.

———. *A Year to Live: How to Live This Year as If It Were Your Last.* New York: Bell Tower, 1997.

Myss, Caroline M., Ph.D. *Why People Don't Heal and How They Can.* New York: Harmony Books, 1997.

Myss, Caroline M., Ph.D., and C. Norman Shealy, M.D. *The Creation of Health: The Emotional, Psychological, and Spiritual Responses That Promote Health and Healing.* New York: Three Rivers Press, 1998.

Naiman, Ingrid. *The Astrology of Healing: Cancer.* Santa Fe, NM: Seventh Ray Press, 1988.

O'Regan, Brendan. "Healing, Remission, and Miracle Cures." *Whole Earth Review* (Winter 1989): 126–135.

Pierrakos, Eva. *The Path of Self-Transformation.* New York: Bantam, 1990.

Rajneesh, Bhagwan Shree. *The Book of Secrets.* Vol. 4. Antelope, OR: Rajneesh Foundation International, 1976.

Rand, William Lee. *Reiki: The Healing Touch.* Southfield, MI: Vision Publications, 1991. Available by calling 800-332-8112.

Rudhyar, Dane. *The Astrology of Personality: A Reformulation of Astrological Concepts and Ideals in Terms of Contemporary Psychology and Philosophy.* Santa Fe, NM: Aurora Press, 1990.

Sanford, Agnes Mary White. *The Healing Light: The Art and Method of Spiritual Healing.* New York: Ballantine, 1990.

Siegel, Bernie S., M.D. *How to Live Between Office Visits: A Guide to Life, Love and Health.* New York: HarperCollins, 1993.

———. *Love, Medicine, & Miracles: Lessons Learned About Self-Healing from a Surgeon's Experience with Exceptional Patients.* New York: Harper & Row, 1986.

———. *Peace, Love, & Healing: Bodymind Communication and the Path to Self-Healing: An Exploration.* New York: Harper & Row, 1989.

Simonton, O. Carl, M.D., Stephanie Matthews-Simonton, and James L.

Creighton. *Getting Well Again: A Step-by-Step, Self-Help Guide to Overcoming Cancer for Patients and Their Families.* Los Angeles, CA: J. P. Tarcher, 1978.

Spangler, David. *Everyday Miracles: The Inner Art of Manifestation.* New York: Bantam, 1996.

———. *The Laws of Manifestation.* Forres, Scotland: Findhorn Foundation, 1975.

Stein, Diane. *Essential Reiki: A Complete Guide to an Ancient Healing Art.* Freedom, CA: Crossing Press, 1995.

The Teaching of Buddha. Tokyo: Bukkyo Dendo Kyokai, 1966.

Thesenga, Susan. *The Undefended Self: Living the Pathwork of Spiritual Wholeness.* 2d ed. Madison, VA: Pathwork Press, 1994.

Trungpa, Chogyam. *Cutting Through Spiritual Materialism.* Boston: Shambhala, 1973.

Wager, Susan, M.D., and Dora Kunz. *A Doctor's Guide to Therapeutic Touch: Enhancing the Body's Energy to Promote Healing.* New York: Perigee/Putnam, 1996.

Wapnick, Kenneth, Ph.D. *A Talk Given on a Course in Miracles: An Introduction.* 4th ed. Roscoe, NY: Foundation for A Course in Miracles, 1996.

Wapnick, Kenneth, Ph.D., and Gloria Wapnick. *Awaken from the Dream.* Roscoe, NY: Foundation for A Course in Miracles, 1995.

Weiss, Brian, M.D. *Many Lives, Many Masters.* New York: Simon & Schuster, 1988.

Woolger, Roger, Ph.D. *Other Lives, Other Selves: A Jungian Psychotherapist Discovers Past Lives.* New York: Doubleday, 1987.

Yogananda, Paramahansa. *Autobiography of a Yogi.* Los Angeles, CA: Self-Realization Fellowship, 1971.

Zelman, Stuart, M.D., and David Bognar. *Human Operators Manual: How Feelings Work: A Psychological Primer.* Hartford, CT: n.p., 1991.

Chapter 9   Cancer and Mortality

American Association of Retired Persons. *Shape Your Health Care Future with Health Care Advance Directives.* Booklet

Callanan, Maggie, and Patricia Kelley. *Final Gifts: Understanding the Special Awareness, Needs, and Communications of the Dying.* New York: Bantam, 1997.

Dass, Ram, and Stephen Levine. *Grist for the Mill*. Rev. ed. Berkeley, CA: Celestial Arts, 1988.

Haylock, Pamela J., R.N., and Carol P. Curtiss, R.N. *Cancer Doesn't Have to Hurt: How to Conquer the Pain Caused by Cancer and Cancer Treatment*. Alameda, CA: Hunter House, 1997.

Lang, Susan S., and Richard B. Pett. *You Don't Have to Suffer: A Complete Guide to Relieving Pain for Patients and Their Families*. New York: Oxford University Press, 1994.

LeShan, Lawrence, Ph.D. *Cancer as a Turning Point: A Handbook for People with Cancer, Their Families, and Health Professionals*. New York: Dutton/Penguin, 1989.

Levine, Stephen. *A Gradual Awakening: An Introduction to Buddhist Meditation*. Garden City, NY: Anchor/Doubleday, 1979.

———. *Guided Meditations, Explorations, and Healings*. New York: Anchor/Doubleday, 1991.

———. *Healing into Life and Death*. New York: Anchor/Doubleday, 1987.

———. *Meetings at the Edge: Dialogues with the Grieving and Dying, the Healing and the Healed*. Garden City, NY: Anchor/Doubleday, 1984.

———. *Who Dies? An Investigation of Conscious Living and Conscious Dying*. New York: Anchor/Doubleday, 1982.

———. *A Year to Live: How to Live This Year as If It Were Your Last*. New York: Bell Tower, 1997.

Marwick, Charles. "Should Physicians Prescribe Prayer for Health? Spiritual Aspects of Well-Being Considered." *Journal of the American Medical Association* 273 (May 24/31, 1995): 1561–62.

Moody, Raymond A., M.D. *The Light Beyond*. New York: Bantam, 1989.

Quill, Timothy E., M.D. *A Midwife Through the Dying Process: Stories of Healing and Hard Choices at the End of Life*. Baltimore, MD: Johns Hopkins University Press, 1996.

Ring, Kenneth. *Healing Toward Omega: In Search of the Meaning of the Near-Death Experience*. New York: William Morrow, 1985.

Vitez, Michael. *Final Choices: Seeking the Good Death*. Philadelphia, PA: Camino Books, 1998.

Zelman, Stuart, M.D., and David Bognar. *Human Operators Manual: How Feelings Work: A Psychological Primer*. Hartford, CT: n.p., 1991.

Subject Index

Personal names appear in a separate index starting on page 297.

Name Index

This index contains all the personal names that appear in the text on pages 1–247, but not those in the Resources sections, pages 248–289.

ALSO FROM DAVID BOGNAR

....

CANCER: Increasing Your Odds for Survival

The Documentary
hosted by Walter Cronkite

CANCER: Increasing Your Odds for Survival is a four hour public
television series hosted by Walter Cronkite. Like this book, it is
divided into four parts: Diagnosis & Empowerment, Treatments,
Mind/Body Interventions, and Spirituality and Mortality. It is
specifically designed to help people survive cancer by providing
an overview of traditional medical treatments and how these can
be supplemented with healing techniques and support methods
for healing cancer.

It is available to purchase for $69.95 plus $5.00 shipping from:

**New Way Productions
PO Box 8241
Manchester, CT 06040
or by calling toll-free 888-307-4482**

For information on related tapes, materials, information, and
cancer links, please visit the website at:

www.cancersurvival.com

*Please send all orders for this videotape direct to the address
above, and do not combine orders or payments with orders for
Hunter House books including reorders for this book.*